Your Body's
BRILLIANT DESIGN

PRAISE FOR KAREN GABLER AND SUSTAINABLE BODY

Mary Kay K., registered nurse/holistic health professional

Sustainable Body is one of the most intelligent and commonsense explanations and demonstrations of the cause of pain and dysfunction. The method gives me the tools to feel better and the support to make much needed, life-affirming lifestyle changes. . . . Pure genius.

Margot C., musician/performer

What I love about Karen's Sustainable Body method is that it's highly effective and the exercises are so enjoyable that I actually want to do them. My body likes them. I feel an "ahhh" of relief when I begin and a "hmmm" of new energy when I finish. They don't take a lot of time, and they work to strengthen me and give me a feeling of well-being for the day. My chronic shoulder pain is reduced or eliminated.

Erin C., critical care nurse

I have noticed that the Sustainable Body routine helps my body work through traumas and achieve a deeper healing than what I had thought possible. Never have I experienced relief that is so profound, lasting, and thorough.

Krista Q., yoga instructor/wellness coach

I came to Karen because I had been experiencing chronic pain radiating from my low back to my hips for years. [I] had seen chiropractors, orthopedics, and physical therapists with fragmented success. . . . [Karen] guides you with a combination of techniques and innate intuition toward an intrinsic alignment of body, mind, and spirit. Months later, I can return to pain-free or close-to- it activity using Karen's Sustainable Body method.

Fran W., photographer/author/professional gardener

I have learned so much about how the human body works, thanks to Karen. Her visual images and cues have helped me to understand the importance of fascia, hydration, and the body's ability to support itself using this misunderstood component of our essential core.

Linda K., camp owner/professional pianist

I had debilitating pain . . . in my foot, and my walking was increasingly compromised. I saw a podiatrist and then a surgeon. Both had a bleak outlook. Karen was optimistic from the start. She worked with the domes of my body, analyzed my gait, and worked at the level of the fascia. I am still amazed that I have regained normal walking ability with little or no discomfort. I can use the elliptical and do floor exercises again. I can take walks and do all the activities I had been forced to give up. I am delighted with this outcome, which is so different from my doctors' pessimistic opinions.

Jerry M., associate professor of engineering

After many restorative sessions in Karen's knowing hands, I am finally doing, at age sixty-eight, what my mother had always told me to do. I am beginning to stand up straight, and I am happy to say that I feel comfortable when I do.

Erica C., PhD student, mother of three

After several years of chronic back pain I had gotten used to viewing my body as problematic. Working with Karen I found a way to reconnect with the inherent strength and wisdom of my body. For the first time, I experience my body as a healthy, whole unit, not as separate problem areas. The Sustainable Body roller routine serves as a daily reminder to reconnect, stabilize, and strengthen my inner core, and when I miss a few days I notice the difference.

PRAISE FROM PRACTITIONERS

Laura H., massage therapist, polarity therapist, Zero Balancer, movement educator

[Sustainable Body] empowers people to take charge of their bodies and make new, informed choices for healthier daily habits. What I continue to learn is that bodywork alone, as potent and healing as it can be, can sometimes generate only temporary change. If we can also identify and work with movement habits that are creating discomfort and dysfunction, day after day, and develop new patterns of moving that draw upon the body's innately intelligent design, we amplify the possibility of lasting change. This kind of "redesigning" of the body is exactly what Karen does in her work. [Sustainable Body] bridges bodywork and movement work in new and skillful ways that facilitate an experience of strength, connection, and wholeness.

Megan G., yoga instructor/dancer

The tangible clarity Karen brings to the understanding of our miraculous bodies, with her elegant explanations and user-friendly exercises, is revelatory to all who it enlightens. Add to that, she is a gifted healer who walks her talk. I personally can't wait to use her book as a reference and tool in my work as a full-time yoga instructor.

Joy F., fitness instructor

[Sustainable Body] is an invaluable resource for fitness professionals such as myself, whose job it is to keep up on the latest trends, teachings, and discoveries. Thanks to Karen, I now more fully understand the interconnectivity and fluidity of the human body and I can pass this on to my clients through improved cueing and explanation. Karen's body of work is important for all of us: yoga teachers, fitness instructors, and all of those dedicated to living their best lives.

Cynthia W., Ortho-Bionomy practitioner/instructor

What I love about Karen's work is that it is a unique creation that allows for strength and support in the body without overworking muscles. The work comes from a place of ease that accounts for an individual's posture and looks deeply into the body, taking its foundation from the breath.

Deborah R., PhD, psychologist

As a psychologist who also treats trauma patients from a mind-body perspective, I've learned a great deal both personally and professionally from Karen's work. At times, it has been extremely uncomfortable emotionally and physically, but I now understand this is part of clearing out the effects of trauma on many different levels in the hopes of repatterning the muscles, fascia, and nervous system itself.

Your Body's
BRILLIANT DESIGN

A REVOLUTIONARY APPROACH
TO RELIEVING CHRONIC PAIN

KAREN M. GABLER

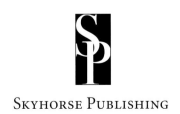

Skyhorse Publishing

Skyhorse Publishing books may be purchased in bulk at special discounts for sales promotion, corporate gifts, fund-raising, or educational purposes. Special editions can also be created to specifications. For details, contact the Special Sales Department, Skyhorse Publishing, 307 West 36th Street, 11th Floor, New York, NY 10018 or info@skyhorsepublishing.com.

Skyhorse® and Skyhorse Publishing® are registered trademarks of Skyhorse Publishing, Inc.®, a Delaware corporation.

Visit our website at www.skyhorsepublishing.com.

10 9 8 7 6 5 4 3 2 1

Library of Congress Cataloging-in-Publication Data is available on file.

Cover design by Jenny Zemanek
Cover illustrations: iStockphoto

Print ISBN: 978–1–5107–1641–4
Ebook ISBN: 978-1-5107-1642-1

Printed in China

Represented by Danielle Burby
Hannigan Salky Getzler Agency
37 West 28th St, 8th Floor
New York, NY 10001

Author's Note

This book presents a point of view and is not meant to be a complete analysis of the role of fascia or its role in pathology. This book combines my thirty-plus years of a hands-on therapy practice working with the bones, fascia, and movement to help myself and my clients embrace the body's brilliant design. This design supports our posture, movements, and our overall health. I would like to share with you my fascination with the alignment of bones, muscles, and fascia and how movement brings them all together. With this fascination, I share with you the role of fascia and the new research on fascia that is helping us understand its importance. The more we understand fascia, the more we can understand its holistic nature. The more we use new imagery that shows us our bodies as whole, interconnected webs of relationships between the parts, we can embrace the wisdom of the architecture within us.

These practices are not intended to replace the services of your physician or provide an alternative to any medical treatment. To reduce the risk of injury, please consult with your doctor before beginning this or any exercise program.

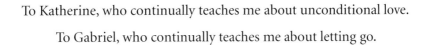

To Katherine, who continually teaches me about unconditional love.

To Gabriel, who continually teaches me about letting go.

Contents

Foreword

In this book, *Your Body's Brilliant Design*, Karen Gabler brings together her thirty-plus years of experience as a hands-on bodyworker, movement educator, yoga practitioner, and teacher to share cutting-edge information and innovative techniques for treating chronic pain. In Karen's book, the lay reader will find an easily comprehensible language along with new images of the human body that will give readers a deeper understanding of the internal architecture of the body and how to move within it with grace and ease. With keen perception and refined anatomical knowledge, Karen brings a precise lens to the inner mechanisms of the body's deepest core and how to use it in everyday life.

I first met Karen through Tom Myers, an advanced Rolfer, who remapped the body's connective tissue, the fascia, into what is now called Anatomy Trains. Her study of fascia, a critically important aspect of human anatomy that has been neglected, opens our eyes to this new paradigm.

Karen and I crossed paths again in a training with Judith Aston, an advanced Rolfer and a brilliant movement educator. We worked together in one of Judith's dyads in which we were taught how to tie our shoes so that the foot can be used for walking in a more optimal way. We found that we shared a common interest and curiosity about the body and how it works. Karen continued to explore and synthesize the foundational support the feet bring to our upright structures, which she shares in this book. Another concept we learned from Judith was how to lengthen the spine in sitting. With Karen's unique lens, she teaches us where in the body this length can be found as well as how to use it.

Karen has created a new marriage of fascia, bones, and movement encompassed under a spiritual umbrella. I have received her work and recommend it to people so they can explore the inner core. Instead of focusing on the outer core or outer sleeve of the body only, Karen's work draws us into the more subtle sensations of the inner core, which begins in the feet, runs up the inseam of the legs, through the pelvis, torso, neck, and head.

Bodyworkers talk about the legs as part of our upright posture, and how the legs are two cylinders, the right and left legs are like hemispheres that continue all the way up to the shoulders. When we look at our clients, we often see them rolled in toward the center line on the vertical axis. After a session with Karen, I could feel these two cylinders being oiled from the legs all the way up to the shoulders. My fascia felt lubricated, which allowed the bones of my skeleton to move in or out freely and in a more efficient way. Her warm touch, welcoming demeanor, and anatomical curiosity allows a client to participate in an active, yet meditative way.

I thank Karen for coming up with this beautiful book, which synthesizes complex anatomical knowledge in such an easy and pleasurable way. She acquaints us with important information about the fascial body that until now had been missing. Not only does she introduce us to the inner architecture of the fascial body, but she also gives people a program they can follow to establish and sustain this inner knowing of the body. This book is a bridge into the new paradigm for relieving chronic pain.

—Yaron Gal Carmel, LCMT, senior faculty
at the Kinesis School of Structural Integration

Introduction:
My Journey into Movement and Stillness

The body and how it moves has always fascinated me. From an early age, movement has been the avenue through which I take in information about the world, learn how to be in it, and take a stand in it. When I was five, my mother signed me up for dance lessons in tap, toe, and ballet. By age seven I was on pointe shoes. In addition to dance, I spent hours in the woods behind my childhood home. One vivid memory I have is of watching water spiders glide over the surface of the babbling brook. I was mesmerized by how effortlessly they moved as their little legs were suspended and yet grounded on the rippling water surface. How did they do that? I would try to copy them as I jumped from rock to rock without falling into the water.

Movement always brought me joy. I trusted my body, so I would take risks. When I was seven, my sister and I were exploring in the woods behind our home. In a clearing, we came upon a large dam with a drop of forty or fifty feet. The dividing line between the calm river with the current swirling as it hit the dam and the steep drop where the water came crashing down onto rocks below was a narrow, concrete ridge. I looked at that ridge and wondered what it would be like to walk across it to the other side. My sister was scared and wanted to turn back, but I wanted to take the challenge. I lowered myself carefully down onto that narrow precipice. Looking down the steep slope of falling water, I realized that if I fell, I likely would not survive. Or if I did, the fall would be serious. I had to balance and trust my body. With focus, determination, and the exhilaration of fear, I walked across to the other side. This brought me the thrill of accomplishment. Once I had done it, my sister followed. We never told our parents what we had done. Now that I am a parent, I think it is better that they did not know.

Finding Stillness

When I was in college, I learned to balance my love of movement with stillness. The stillness I had found being in the woods as a child was now replaced with learning Transcendental Meditation. After college, I lived and worked in Australia and then began a yearlong journey around the world alone with a backpack, no itinerary, and a large dose of courage. At one point along the journey, I landed in India. While there, I was led to a ten-day silent Vipassana meditation retreat in the same location the Buddha himself had been enlightened more than 2,500 years ago. Under the guidance of one of the foremost teachers in the lineage of this kind of meditation, I learned to sit still and observe the constantly moving sensations in my body in order to clear my mind. This retreat was extremely challenging for me. To sit still without moving was, at times, excruciating. Little did I know that I was in the process of observing the theme of my life: movement and stillness in the body.

Discovering Bodywork

After a year of teaching in Australia, a year of world travel, and several years editing textbooks in large publishing houses in Boston, my life hit a huge bump. Something was off; I was out of sync with myself. To help me navigate this bumpy road, I started seeing a Jungian therapist. As part of my therapy, she suggested I get some hands-on therapy, or bodywork. I took her advice.

The first practitioner I saw for a hands-on bodywork session was a gifted Alexander Technique teacher. The Alexander Technique is a practical method that uses awareness to reeducate the body's neuromuscular system. One can learn to use this overall awareness, to let go of tension patterns and create new patterns of ease. This practitioner had me lie on her massage table as she worked. I had no idea what she was doing with her hands, but whatever it was, I felt transformed. I got up from the table after the session with a sensation of lightness, expansion, and ease. All the rocky bumps in my life looked different from my new body's perspective. My curiosity was piqued.

My therapist then recommended I see another practitioner of hands-on therapy. This person practiced a modality called Zero Balancing. Zero Balancing is a hands-on body–mind therapy that uses skilled touch to address the relationships between energy and structure within the body. The practitioner uses his/her hands to create points of balance in specific bones and joints around which the body can relax and reorganize. Its objective is to help a person's system rebalance in order to promote greater health and well-being. Under this practitioner's skilled hands, a profound thing happened to me. During this one session, my body went from being all disjointed and disconnected to being connected into an effortless alignment from the inside out. I stood up from the table feeling solid, rooted, aligned, and suspended simultaneously. My life and its many problems looked different from this aligned place.

From these two hands-on therapy experiences, I knew I wanted to learn how to use touch to create this feeling in the body and share it with others. My life took a dramatic turn. I did not know it then, but I had found my life's passion: how to use conscious touch to align the whole body, mind, and spirit.

Learning Bodywork

My journey into the world of practicing hands-on therapy began with learning Zero Balancing, the technique that had helped me experience such profound alignment. Zero Balancing was developed by Fritz Frederick Smith, MD, in the early 1970s. It addresses the whole skeleton by focusing on specific foundation joints in the pelvis, spine, hips, and feet that are designed to provide stability and transmit forces through the body. Unlike freely movable joints, such as the elbow or shoulder joints that are mostly used for movement and locomotion, foundation joints have a small range of motion and depend on the quality of the ligaments within them for balance and ease of movement. When foundation joints are stuck, the body's whole musculoskeletal system goes out of balance. We are not aware that this is happening. Instead of correcting themselves, these joints remain stuck and the body starts to compensate around the imbalance. Following a protocol that typically lasts thirty to forty-five minutes, the Zero Balancing practitioner uses his/her hands to evaluate these joints for tissue-held tension, joint play, and quality of motion, and then treats them by utilizing finger pressure and gentle traction to balance the joints. When these joints are balanced, formerly stuck physical, mental, and spiritual issues can be released and new patterns of alignment and balance from deep within the body's structure can emerge.

A colleague described a Zero Balancing session this way: "It is a massage with your clothes on, therapy without talking, and an altered state without meditation or mind-altering substances." Zero Balancing has had profound effects on my alignment, my health, and my healing.

By studying Zero Balancing directly with Dr. Fritz Smith himself and his protégé, Jim McCormick, I have learned that skilled touch, perhaps the oldest and still most reliable healing modality we possess, can be used to create motion and stillness in the body in a gentle, unobtrusive way. When motion and stillness are balanced, there is a natural extension into the body and the mind that allows healing and more optimal physical, emotional, and spiritual health.

My study of Zero Balancing led me to massage school, which gave me traditional training in anatomy and physiology. As I was being trained and licensed to practice massage therapy, a guest lecturer came to our school and introduced me to the concept of fascia. Fascia is the body's seamless web of connective tissue that weaves in and throughout muscles, bones, organs, and cells. Just as I was drawn to how the skeleton connects as a whole, I was drawn to fascia and how it connects the whole body. Yet my anatomy and physiology textbooks from massage school did not show this tissue. I wanted to know more about this responsive, adaptable tissue and how it creates our alignment and posture.

Once I graduated from massage school, I delved into Structural Integration training, which came out of the lineage of Dr. Ida Rolf.[1] Fascia is very strong and very flexible, yet at the time of Dr. Rolf it was not even considered as a tissue that determined

---

1 Dr. Rolf was one of the pioneers in the field of hands-on and movement therapies and contributed significantly to the holistic view of the body. She brought fascia into the lexicon of the body–mind therapy movement. In the 1950s, she developed a technique called Structural Integration, better known as Rolfing. Structural Integration manually releases physical tensions in the fascia that prevent balanced alignment, or optimal posture. At the time Dr. Rolf was developing her method, the common thought was that soft tissue could not hold change.

the structure of the body. Bone-setting (osteopathy and chiropractic) was the only treatment for structure that was thought to be effective. Because of Rolf's work, people began to view the body differently. Dr. Rolf taught us that the fascia holds the alignment and the posture of the body.

One of Dr. Rolf's first students, psychologist Dr. Bill Williams, expanded Rolfing to include the psychological implications of changes in the fascia; he called the practice SOMA Neuromuscular Integration. By studying these techniques, I learned how to align the fascia using Structural Integration principles from Dr. Rolf and how to support my clients in those changes using the psychological principles of Dr. Williams.

Fascial Release

Working with connective tissue or fascia takes different training and skills than working with muscles, as is done in massage. In order to manually remodel the connective tissue, the practitioner needs to use a different style of contact, or deep touch, called fascial release. Fascia is made up of strong collagen fibers and a matrix of ground substance that is malleable. The ground substance is like gelatin. Gelatin gets solid and hard when you put it in the refrigerator, and it gets soft and liquid when you heat it up. The ground substance in fascia gets hard and thick when it is under strain, but gets soft and liquid with deep touch and multi-vector movement. When this deep touch is applied with a specific direction, pressure, and speed, the ground substance melts into a more liquid state and the collagen fibers lengthen and slide over each other more easily. Fascia that has been deformed by injury, surgery, poor posture, or disuse can be released and remodeled. Using touch and stretch, the new dynamically fluid environment enables the muscles, ligaments, tendons, bones, nerves, and even individual cells within the fascial system to realign and reset themselves.

Discovering the Body's Core

As I incorporated my skills in touching bone with my skills in touching fascia into my private sessions, my work expanded. I was led to a new teacher in the world of fascia,

Thomas Myers, who developed an all-encompassing map of the fascial web.[2] Myers mapped the fascial web into twelve myofascial meridians (vertical lines of fascia and muscles) that help us understand how the fascia is connected, and how it is used for movement.[3] This work dramatically changed my perspective on how I looked at the body.

Imagine the individual myofascial meridians as three-dimensional sets of muscles and connective tissues that form the entire volume of the musculoskeletal system. The first three lines run more or less straight up and down the body—front, back, and sides. Several other lines wind through and across the first three lines, affecting movement and posture directly or indirectly. One myofascial meridian especially caught my attention: the Deep Front Line. This line, running from the arches of the feet to the crown of the head, is the deepest and takes up more volume and space in the body than any of the other lines. Its counterpart, the Deep Back Line,[4] also begins in the arches of the feet and runs up the legs, but then departs from the Deep Front Line and runs up the back of the body. It seems likely that these fascial guidewires form the Vertical Core of the body that allows our posture to be effortless.

When these fascial guidewires are not in balance, this is the perfect storm for chronic pain to develop. By restoring the proper function of and connection to this deep fascia using touch, breath, and movement, many issues of chronic pain can be treated and resolved, and many issues can be prevented.

Back to Movement

Movement is key to integrating the changes made in the bones and the fascia. While the hands-on bodywork can help you discover your deep inner core alignment, it is movement that will help you embody that alignment in everyday life.

---

2 Myers, Thomas. 2014. *Anatomy Trains: Myofascial Meridians for Manual and Movement Therapists, 3rd Edition,* Churchill Livingstone.

3 Myers exposed these myofascial meridians in dissection by altering the usual dissection method: turning the scalpel sideways to create vertical connections rather than separation, which opened up a whole new paradigm of myofascia that inspires many manual and movement therapists.

4 The Deep Back Line was uncovered by Yaron Gal Carmel, a teacher on the faculty at Myers's school and one of his protégés.

Finding your Vertical Core alignment is not about being in a particular held posture, like sitting up straight with shoulders back. Your Vertical Core is found through a process of working with the natural curves of the spine and involves letting go of habitual movement patterns and listening to what feels effortless. We cannot "think" ourselves into better posture. We need to *feel* the effortlessness of good posture to make it sustainable. I began to experiment with how to make a connection between dynamic stability and elastic movement to find a user-friendly way for you to embody the Vertical Core and sustain a new posture more consciously. I call this Sustainable Body.

Growing Sustainable Body

Sustainable Body Training grew out of an understanding that stuck, tense fascia, especially at the foundation and semi-foundation joints, can be realigned and rehydrated *and* that breath and movement can sustain that alignment and hydration. Many fascial fitness methods[5] address the importance of hydrating fascia. But they do not address alignment through the holistic lens of this deep fascial core that is integral to a Sustainable Body.

In addition to keeping the fascia healthy and fit, you must understand how to keep connected with its natural alignment and balance. I discovered that by lying on a 36-inch soft foam roller, I could make the necessary neurofascial connections to the Vertical Core and the center of gravity in my body efficiently and relatively quickly.

I decided to do an experiment. I stopped my yoga practice, weight training, and running. Instead, I continued my walking and lying on the soft roller, practicing the specific movements that activated the center of gravity through breath and the Vertical Core fascial guidewires. I did this for seven months straight. I began to teach the routine to my clients and in workshops, and people noticed that it made a difference in their strength and alignment.

---

5 Fascial Fitness, developed out of Germany by Dr. Robert Schleip, and Sue Hitzmann's MELT Method are examples.

One day, I went kayaking with a friend who was an avid athlete. I had not been kayaking for a couple of years. When I lifted the kayak into the water, I was struck by how light it felt. We headed out to the ocean and came upon a narrow passageway between two rocks. I steered my kayak between the rocks and realized the current was stronger than I expected. I focused on using my center of gravity and the Vertical Core guidewires I had been training into my body on the roller. My lower body was connected to its center of gravity, and my upper body felt squarely on top of the lower body because it felt connected through the vertical guidewires. I navigated through the rocks and came out on the other side. My friend was impressed by how well I had done. I realized how strong and centered I felt; I was using the power of my fascia and transmitting forces through it more efficiently than I ever had before. I knew I was onto something!

The synthesis of my knowledge of bones, fascia, and movement has grown into what I call Sustainable Body Training. This method is based on how the new anatomy of fascia connects every single part of the body into a whole. It combines:

1) my knowledge of bones and aligning the skeleton at the key foundational joints that balance the whole skeleton and connect it to the body's energetic core;
2) my knowledge of fascial release and aligning the whole fascial web by connecting to the body's deep myofascial core; and
3) how to use breath and subtle balancing movements to embody this alignment.

It is my premise that if you focus on connecting to the center of gravity in the pelvis with breath, what I call the Core Hug (see Chapter 9), and activate the deep Vertical Core fascial guidewires with movement (see Chapter 10), your whole body reconnects to the architecture designed for alignment and suspension. You can create a new posture from within. When you reconnect to the body's true core, you have an opportunity to rediscover the body's brilliant design and how to use it to relieve chronic pain.

Prologue:
Sustainable Body

Every day I meet people with chronic pain who have sought help and tried many treatments without success. They have exhausted their resources and feel hopeless that they will never be free of pain.

What's the key that many doctors, physical therapists, massage therapists and fitness educators are missing?

The fascia.

Fascia is the body's seamless web of connective tissue that weaves in and throughout muscles, bones, organs, and cells. It connects us from head to toe, from skin to bone. This resilient biological fabric surrounds every muscle, bone, organ, and each individual cell. Since the body and everything in it is connected by this tissue, it is important to look at where fascia is pulled, strained, disconnected, and misaligned. When the fascia is strained or pulled out of alignment, it pulls muscles, bones, and joints out of alignment and causes symptoms of chronic pain. That shoulder pain you are experiencing could be the result of fascia pulled out of alignment when you injured your foot twenty years ago. (More on that in Part 2.)

Did you know that your body is designed to keep you out of pain? In fact, it is brilliantly designed to live in alignment and ease. The only way to do this is to connect to the fascia: the tissue that connects everything together.

How?

Taking charge of your own healing begins with understanding your body's brilliant design. The human body is organized in an intelligent way to stabilize and move from the fascia's center of gravity and inner core. With this book, you will learn how to connect to the center of gravity in your body using your breath and how to connect to your inner core using subtle movement. Using these connections and this wisdom of your own body, you can learn to sustain whole-body alignment in your everyday life and live pain-free. In doing so, you will be living in your own Sustainable Body.

How to Use this Book

Part 1 introduces you to the concepts you will learn in this book and answers questions like: What is Sustainable Body training? How is it different from what I have tried before? Is it for me? You will learn where your true core resides and that a soft foam roller may be the key to finding it.

In Part 2, you will delve into the fascinating science of fascia and how our bodies are brilliantly designed to keep us out of pain. You will learn about how the body uses tension and compression forces to balance itself effortlessly, and how fascia even has its own nervous system! You will then explore each component of Sustainable Body Training: the center of the fascial web and how to use breath to find it, how to activate and train the deep inner core, and how to align the domes and fans of your body's architecture from the center out. I will walk you through a few exercises in breath and subtle movement so you can start to feel the difference for yourself.

Part 3 takes you through some of the latest research on breath and movement and how we need to change the way we exercise in order to combat chronic pain.

The full Sustainable Body Training Sequence in Part 4 gives you a step-by-step guide to training alignment of the fascia through breath and from the inside out, complete with full-color photographs of each step.

I hope you enjoy discovering your body's brilliant design and how by connecting to it, training it, and embodying it you can live in alignment, balance, strength, flexibility, and ease. We are not designed to be in chronic pain. In fact, we are designed to live an aligned and buoyant life! Are you ready to join me on the journey into the architecture that already lives within you?

Please visit my website at www.gablersustainablebody.com and feel free to write me at karen@gablersustainablebody.com about your experiences and if you have any questions. I look forward to hearing about your journey to discover your own body's brilliant design!

Karen M. Gabler, LMT

PART ONE

OVERVIEW

"We do not have a health care crisis. We have a self-care crisis."[6]

—Michaelle Edwards

Did you know there are two types of pain? Acute pain and chronic pain. When you break a leg or badly sprain an ankle, the cause of acute pain is usually clear. The pain is associated with a one-time event or trauma and you know why you are experiencing intense pain. This type of pain can be treated with drugs, surgery, and rest. The treatment offered by doctors when we experience acute pain such as a car accident, migraines, or an appendicitis attack is important and critical. As the acute injury is treated and starts to heal, pain usually subsides.

Chronic pain is another matter. Chronic pain can often be mysterious, and you may be unsure why you have the pain at all. For example, when you sit for long hours at the office or drive in your car, your back starts to hurt. The daily walk you enjoy becomes difficult because after an hour your hip begins to hurt. The foot pain that used to come on every couple of months now occurs frequently. Or the shoulder that bothered you only when you reached into the back seat of your car is now extremely painful after that challenging workout at the gym.

Chronic pain is not so clear cut. Doctors do not know how to treat this kind of pain as effectively because they are not aware of the cause of the chronic pain. In this book, you will learn why you have chronic pain and where it comes from (hint: the fascia).

Using the same methods for treating acute pain, doctors prescribe medications that reduce inflammation and stop the signals of pain. Yet pain relief is often temporary

---

6 Edwards, Michaelle. 2011. *YogAlign: Pain-Free Yoga from Your Inner Core.* Hihimanu Press.

or minimal. In this book, you'll learn why medication does not work to relieve chronic pain.

If medication does not work, doctors will prescribe physical therapy programs that give you exercises to stretch or strengthen certain muscles. In this book, you will not learn specific exercises for specific muscles. Instead you will learn how to use the body as one continuous muscle system.

Some programs require heavy workouts to stay out of pain. Not this one. You will learn simple and gentle movements for the whole body that can relieve chronic pain and sustain that relief.

As a last resort, doctors often prescribe surgery to relieve the pain. In this book, you will learn ways to prevent surgery, as well as prepare for a more successful pre-surgery and post-surgery experience.

A New Way to Think About Chronic Pain

The program in this book, the Sustainable Body Training method, uses a radically different approach to treating chronic pain. This training is based on decades of groundbreaking and little-known research on the only tissue in the human body that connects each and every part: *fascia*. Fascia is the body's seamless web of connective tissue that unifies all the parts as it weaves in and throughout muscles, bones, organs, and cells. Without fascia to contain and shape the body, you would fall into a heap on the ground. Without fascia, muscles could not connect to bones, bones would not be able to support you, and joints would not be able to work at all.

Western anatomy has focused on breaking the body down into parts and seeing movement as individual muscles that attach to bones which move us using mechanical leverage. This muscle–bone concept presented in anatomy textbooks separates movement into discrete functions, which gives us a mechanical model of the human body and its movement. But we are not robots. What has been missing, and what this book introduces to you, is the tissue that unites all the parts: the connective tissue, or fascia.

Not only will you learn about fascia, but you will also learn how fascia just may be the cause of your chronic pain. The body is designed to use the fascia to sustain its alignment, stability, and fluid movement. Unfortunately, the fascia can get deformed by injury, surgery, poor posture, or repetitive movement. When your fascia is out of alignment, your muscles, bones, and joints get out of alignment. The fascia then loses its fluidity and becomes stuck and dehydrated. Movement becomes restricted and limited. As a result, you feel stiff and sore. Chronic pain becomes the norm. In this book, you will learn how to use your body's fascial design to create more alignment, better posture, more strength, and greater flexibility. And, you will not have to follow traditional exercise programs to do it!

You will be introduced to the new anatomy of fascia using illustrations that help you visualize how to use your body's architecture. The power of the imagination or mental imagery has been documented as a way to train the brain and the nervous system. When you visualize a movement, your brain sends signals to the muscles involved and the muscles activate. This book includes photographs and illustrations that help you envision some of the complex anatomical concepts presented in this book. When you see the design that resides within you, you are more likely to manifest it. Envisioning your body's design can be your first step toward freedom from chronic pain.

CHAPTER 1

WHAT IS SUSTAINABLE BODY?

Sustainable Body training is unique. It addresses the whole body and teaches you how to activate your deep inner core, which supports the body from the inside out. In addition, it gives you a way to sustain that connection on your own in daily life.

Did you know that you have both an inner core and an outer core[7]? Most of the time when people talk about the "core," they are talking about the outer core muscles. The outer core is designed for movement, while the inner core is designed for foundational support, balance, and posture. The inner core is made up of deep muscles and fascia—the key substance we will be exploring together in this book. It is important to know how to use the inner core. When the inner core is trained, there is a balance between the inner and outer core. As a result, you are more aligned and movement is more efficient. A lot of people overtrain the outer core, which weakens the inner core. This makes optimal posture almost impossible to sustain. Knowing the difference between what the inner core feels like and what the outer core feels like is the key to finally maintaining healthy posture and alleviating chronic pain. This book will teach you how to do that. Once you feel the difference, you will be able to start relieving your own chronic pain.

What Makes this Approach Different?

Many approaches address movement muscles of the outer core and neglect to train the inner core muscles as a whole. This is because movement muscles are easier to identify and train. When movement muscles and joints are out of alignment, you can feel and correct them. For example, a physical therapist might treat your rotator cuff injury in the

---

7 In Structural Integration and Fascial Research Society circles the outer core is known as the outer sleeve.

shoulder by working with the shoulder, or your carpal tunnel by working with your wrist. It is standard protocol to treat where the symptom is manifesting.

But what gives support to the wrist is the alignment of the shoulder. What supports the alignment of the shoulder is determined by the alignment and connection to the inner core—a more subtle concept that you will explore in this book. The inner core gives the body its foundational support. This deep, inner foundational core is what gives the movement joints their stability from the inside out. Movement muscles in the wrist or shoulder may scream out in pain and demand your attention, whereas the inner core is more silent. When your inner core goes out of alignment, it doesn't correct itself. Movement muscles try to compensate for this inner weakness and end up in pain. It's hard to tell when the inner core is out of alignment because it is under your conscious awareness. An out-of-whack shoulder you can feel. A misaligned, disconnected inner core you cannot.

Until the inner core is addressed, movement joints do not have a place to stabilize from. They will keep going out. If you continue to treat the symptom, you will never address the cause. And the cause is usually in your body's foundation—the inner core.

What can realign the inner core? Conscious, subtle movement. Many movement teachers are trying to do that. Pilates aims to stabilize the core. Yoga does this as well. What makes my method different is that you are consistently treating the inner core as a whole using very subtle movements. This training, when practiced and done prior to a Pilates, yoga or fitness routine, enables your body to remain aligned and balanced as you move. This is the part that's usually missing, since we lack a deep understanding of what the inner core truly is.

How Do You Train the Inner Core?

How do you activate and strengthen the inner core? By using a soft foam roller. A roller is a thirty-six-inch cylinder made of soft foam.[8] I highly recommend that you invest in a roller to gain the maximum benefit from this program. You lay your spine vertically along the roller, then engage in specific movements of your extremities. When doing so,

8 I recommend OPTP's Pro-RollerTM Soft model, available at www.optp.com.

you must use the inner core to maintain balance on the roller. A multidimensional activation of the inner core takes place.

The intricate balancing that you experience on the roller is a whole-body experience that is often being missed when you lie on the floor or engage in many other fitness routines. The inner core might be getting trained in parts, but not as a whole.

Training the inner core needs to come first, because it is closest to the deeper parts of the body—closest to the body's center of gravity; closest to its vertical axis. Because it is so deep in the body, you cannot feel it when it goes out. It is subtle. You must train it by paying close attention.

Inner core training:

–is subtle

–is mindful—paying close attention to the sensations deep in your body

–must be well-placed—positioning yourself well before you move determines ease of movement and effectiveness of training

The roller is key to activating those subtle connections to the inner core using small movements. This type of subtle movement training gets missed in practices like yoga, Pilates, fitness training, and physical therapy. You may have noticed that many others have discovered the power of using a roller. Rollers are now often seen in gyms and exercise studios and are being used to release muscles and fascia. That is all good, but instead of working with just releasing muscles and fascia, this training is working within the fascial paradigm of the body's guidewires that make up the true inner core. That is what makes my approach different.

In this book, you will learn how to use the soft foam roller to do breath training and subtle movement and balancing exercises designed to train your inner core (see Part 4).

IMPORTANT ROLLER NOTES:

1. It is important to use a soft roller instead of a hard roller. Why? Because the inner core needs to yield into support. If the roller is too hard, the body cannot yield enough and the training of the inner core is missed. If you do use a hard roller, please lay a thick towel, blanket, or yoga mat over it.

2. The roller is not a good fit for everyone. Please see "Precautions and Contraindications" in Part 4 to see if a roller is right for you.

3. If for any reason you cannot use the roller, inner core training can happen on the floor. A roller is simply the most efficient way to get there.

The focus on deep inner core alignment, which is misunderstood in many circles, is what sets Sustainable Body apart from other approaches. Knowing where the true core resides is key to addressing every aspect of whole body health: posture, alignment, ease of movement, and chronic pain. When you learn about your architecture and how fascia connects this architecture throughout the whole body, you begin to understand your body in a new way. When you perform the breathing and the movement routine on the soft foam roller, you learn to embody this architecture from the inside out.

Sustainable Body Difference

Sustainable Body	Massage Therapy, Chiropractic Therapy, Physical Therapy, etc.
Through conscious touch, subtle movement, and guided anatomical visualization, Sustainable Body connects you to the body's center of gravity and aligns the inner core as a whole. In addition, you learn how to sustain your alignment and live pain-free.	These therapies are often temporary solutions with few lasting benefits. They often address only the symptom and not the cause of pain. They compartmentalize problems and miss opportunities to address the body's center of gravity and the whole inner core, which, when not activated, is the cause of most chronic pain. They also lack prescriptive guidance in how to change postural habits. They do not teach you how to remain in alignment and sustain a pain-free lifestyle.

Architecture of the Inner Core

Sustainable Body is a combination of the knowledge and application of your body's deep inner wisdom. In Part 2 you will learn about the components of your body's brilliant architecture that keep it balanced, vibrant, and healthy. These components are:

Fascia: The body uses fascia to communicate the balance between the bones, muscles, and joints. We use our fascia to hold ourselves up, balance and align us, and negotiate the stresses and strains of life. Read more about it in Chapter 5.

Tensegrity: The body holds itself up using balanced suspension. Tensegrity structures are efficient and adaptive and may help us understand how connected our musculoskeletal system is in new and important ways. Read more about it in Chapter 6.

The Neurofascial System: New research discovered that fascia has a body-wide signaling system that functions like a nervous system, yet is separate and unique in its abilities. This is because specialized sensory nerves that reside mostly in fascia send massive amounts of communication throughout the body with little input from the central nervous system or the brain. Read more about it in Chapter 7.

The Center of Gravity: The human body organizes itself around a single point: the center of gravity, deep in the pelvis. This point is the center of the fascial web. I call this center the Core Hug. Without this signal from the body's center, the body has a challenging time organizing itself for alignment and balance. When you connect to this place within you, the fascial web organizes itself more efficiently. Read more about how to connect to the Core Hug using breath in Chapter 9.

The Vertical Core/Inner Core[9]: Since we are vertical structures, in addition to this center of gravity in the pelvis, the body also organizes around a vertical line. It is essential to know about the four fascial guidewires that run from the arches of your feet to the top of your spine and form your deep inner core of support. These are the fascial guidewires that allow

---

9 I use both terms, "inner core" and "vertical core," interchangeably in this book.

your posture to be effortless. When these fascial guidewires are not in balance, this is the perfect storm for chronic pain to develop. Read more about it in Chapter 10.

Domes and Fans: There are architectural wonders throughout your body that take the shape of domes and fans. It is important to connect these domes and fans to the center of gravity and the Vertical Core in order to feel whole-body alignment. Read more about them in Chapter 12.

Sustainable Body is a method to help you rediscover your body's natural alignment, learn to live in that alignment, and therefore relieve many chronic pain issues. It is a training to sustain alignment over the long term based on how the new anatomy of fascia connects every single part of the body into a whole. If you focus on connecting to the center of gravity in the pelvis with breath and activate the deep Vertical Core fascial guidewires with movement, you can connect to the body's innate wisdom. When the architecture of the deep inner core is aligned and then activated, not only does your fascia and the bones within it balance themselves, but you begin to align from the inside out. This allows you to truly sustain alignment as a way of life, not as a one-time exercise or bodywork session.

Sustainable Body is unique in the way that it not only uses the cutting-edge science and wisdom of fascia to teach you how to align yourself, but it also sets you on a lifelong path of sustaining that alignment and living without pain.

The answers lie within you. Let this method be the key to unlocking them.

CHAPTER 2

IS SUSTAINABLE BODY FOR ME?

Is Sustainable Body for you? In a word, yes. Whether you are young or old, athletic or sedentary, like to exercise or do not at all, people from all walks of life can benefit from reconnecting to the body's center of gravity and its vertical inner core. Athletes, fitness buffs, yoga and Pilates teachers, and dancers experience chronic pain. You would think that because they are fit, strong, and flexible, chronic pain would not be an issue, but this is not always the case. Often the outer core is well trained, yet the inner core is weak or disconnected. This causes tension and strain patterns in the movement muscles and jeopardizes joint alignment and balance. People who are less fit, older, have had surgery, or do not follow a regular exercise routine also experience chronic pain due to the lack of connection to the inner core. Chronic pain can be experienced no matter your age, fitness level, or lifestyle.

Aging

Let's look at aging. The older we get, the tendency to experience chronic pain is more likely. When older patients complain of chronic pain to their doctors, the doctor's answer is often that nothing can be done and that the symptom of pain is because you are getting older. I don't buy into this line of thinking. Chronic pain is a result of repetitive movements, postures, and dysfunctional breathing patterns that develop in the fascia over time, not aging or muscle tension. It is true that as we age the fascia is dehydrating. This is part of the life process. Those wrinkles we see in the skin are a result of our fascia drying out and the accumulation of life experiences that can cause stress to get stuck in the fascia surrounding our internal organs. Aging skin keeps the beauty, cosmetic, and surgery businesses going strong with all the new wrinkle treatments, tummy tucks, and face-lifts. Accumulated stress in the organs can also lead to chronic pain. Those who are aging have just had more time to develop and form poor postural and breathing patterns, which result in joint damage and tissue degeneration.

Even though we cannot reverse the aging process in the fascia, we can slow it down. It is never too late to reconnect to the body's brilliant architecture, no matter how challenged it has been. It still resides within us. The benefits of reconnecting to our natural breathing patterns and the body's center of gravity, retraining our inner core, and rehydrating our fascia from the inside out can be done at any age. Because the subtle movement exercises in the Sustainable Body Training sequence are kind and gentle for the body, people of any age or fitness level can do them. It may take longer to realign and rehydrate a joint that has degenerated, but it is possible. In addition, when we realign and reconnect to how the body uses its natural support system and rehydrate the fascia from there, we are able to take the compression and shear out of joints, muscles, and bones and prevent further damage.

Sedentary lifestyle

Do you sit in front of a computer for much of the day? Does your job involve a long commute by car? Do you spend much of your day using a handheld device like a smartphone? When you finally take a break, do you watch television or a movie on your device sitting slumped on the couch? Unfortunately, our present lifestyles in the Western world ask the human body to stay in positions for which it was not designed. For thousands of years, people lived in natural settings that involved hunting and the gathering of food. As civilization advanced and machines were invented to do much of the work, we moved away from natural movements. Today, many people living in cultures where everyday movements involve walking, carrying things on the head, and squatting instead of sitting still perform natural movements, and the inner core architecture of their bodies is not lost (see more about functional movement in Chapter 15). Today, in the Western world, we sit more than ever before, glued to our computers and digital devices that keep us further and further away from natural movements in our everyday lives. No wonder chronic pain is an epidemic!

Sitting in the same position creates strain throughout the body's fascial fabric, as the body's weight compresses joints and muscles. Fascia will take on the shape we are in. If we are hunched over a computer, the fascia gets the message of strain and tension. We lose our connection to the inner core that holds us up. Our fascia tries to hold up the heavy head using smaller movement muscles at the back of the neck and shoulders. These muscles are not designed to hold up your fifteen-pound head. Chronic neck and upper back pain is the result. As we sit, the low back stays in a rounded position for hours at a time. The fascia in the low back is in constant strain as it tries to figure out how to hold you up without the right support coming from the inner core.

The stresses of work and life can also wreak havoc on the nerves and manifest in shallow breathing. As a result, tension builds throughout the body. The nervous system remains in constant fight-or-flight mode and loses its ability to move into the rest-and-digest phase that is necessary for balance. If we learn to become aware of these signals before they scream at us, we can stop the cycle of chronic pain. We can do this by using the center of gravity, breathing from the inner core, resetting our Vertical Core alignment, and rebalancing our autonomic nervous system.

Athletes, runners, dancers, yogis, and fitness buffs

Other populations affected by chronic pain are athletes, runners, dancers, and those who practice yoga, Pilates, and other forms of fitness. These groups use the body daily to do movement and manage tension and compression forces in the fascia. If the body's alignment is compromised or one is doing repetitive movements over and over in misalignment, the fascia is straining and pulling muscles, bones, and joints out of alignment.

Many yoga and exercise positions put the body in the same position as our chair-sitting position, which creates some of the same tension patterns. A pose performed with rounded shoulders and a rounded spine is not necessarily healthy. Without conscious awareness and activation of your inner core of fascia, you may reinforce poor postures and breathing patterns. Thus, pain and injury are common. Similarly, when exercise is practiced at higher temperatures, the muscles can become so relaxed that the signal that warns the body that the stretch is too much is bypassed. As a result, the stretch goes into the ligaments and tendons, which are fascia, and damage occurs. Have you noticed that most injuries occur in the fascia? We rarely experience a torn muscle. What is more common is a sprained ligament or a torn tendon.

For anyone who practices or teaches fitness and to prevent injuries, it is important to align and stabilize the inner core before engaging in any exercise routine.

Performers: musicians, singers, actors

Musicians, singers, and actors are another group that can benefit from more aligned and healthy fascia. Musicians often adjust their posture to the shape of an instrument. Many performers complain of strain and pain from repetitive movements. Singers and actors need to breathe fully, stand for long hours, and use their bodies under stressful conditions. It is important for performers to connect to the center of gravity and inner core alignment, as well as rehydrate the fascia. A result is that the body is used more efficiently and bounces back from the stress and strain caused by the repetitive movements.

Day-to-day living

No matter what lifestyle you lead, it is important to know how to align and rehydrate the fascia so that muscles, bones, joints, and organs have the space they need to communicate and stay healthy. Fascia is the body-wide communication system that holds the spaces in the body. Hydrated fascia is the spatial medicine the body needs so that each and every part is nourished and replenished on a daily basis. Dehydrated fascia cannot communicate as efficiently as hydrated fascia. When fascia cannot communicate well, our everyday movements, such as sitting, standing, and walking, become less efficient. When fascia communicates well, everyday movement becomes easier. Our bodies take on natural movements with grace and fluidity because our fascia is doing the job it was meant to do. You can learn to use the architecture of fascia as an avenue out of chronic pain and as a sustainable path to a pain-free life.

MY SUSTAINABLE BODY STORY: LINDA K.

"I felt tightness and tension melt away from my bones, and when I looked in the mirror I was amazed at how tall and upright I looked.

I felt connected and solid through my whole torso. What was particularly noticeable was that my feet felt wider and more supportive of my legs and hips. My shoulders and neck released during the session, so I looked and felt taller and more graceful. The stooped over posture was gone.

The length and strength I feel after the session lasts. I notice the times when I am "collapsing," because my body has experienced a new way and wants to correct my old habits. More and more I am naturally walking, sitting, [and] moving in a supported and integrated way. Not only do I notice this, but my friends and family comment on it, and that feels great."

Delving deeper

By educating yourself about your body's architecture and how fascia connects this architecture within you, you will be able to access the natural alignment of your body. When you use this intelligent design properly, the body can heal itself from chronic pain and injury. In fact, it is designed so well that you have the architecture within your fascia and bones to create alignment and balance and to bounce back from the stresses and strains of life. You have the power to realign and put space back into your joints and dissolve bone spurs.

Once you understand how your body is designed to keep you out of pain, you can then learn how to embody this design using breath and movement. When you perform the movement routine in Part 4 with mindful awareness, you will learn to embody this architecture so you are empowered to live a life without pain. When you better understand why chronic pain *actually* happens, you can begin to effectively treat it from the inside out.

In Part 2, we'll delve deeper into the wisdom of your body's architecture and discover how the body uses this architecture to prevent and treat chronic pain.

PART TWO

YOUR BODY'S BRILLIANT DESIGN

"The human body is the best work of art."

—Jess C. Scott, author, artist

CHAPTER 3

A HOLISTIC APPROACH TO CHRONIC PAIN

We are a nation in chronic pain. Out of 238 million American adults, 100 million live in chronic pain. In Judy Foreman's groundbreaking book, *A Nation in Pain*, she states, "When chronic pain goes on for long periods of time and is inadequately treated, it undermines the body and the mind."[10] Chronic pain can be viewed as a disease in its own right; in fact, it may be one of the nation's most serious health crises and is costing us hundreds of billions of dollars. Foreman was astonished by how little doctors know about pain and how to treat it, and how our health care system rewards doctors for interventions like surgery and injections that may or may not work and penalizes doctors for taking time to talk to their patients.

Foreman's book is an in-depth and well-researched account that clearly lays out scientific research on everything from neurobiology to public policy, from prescription painkillers to new surgeries for chronic pain patients. It appears that Foreman's book covers most of the research on pain. It even devotes a chapter to fair-minded assessments of alternative medicine techniques. Foreman points out that research supports exercise as a treatment for chronic pain, but "no one knows exactly why" it works or exactly what kind of exercise helps the most.[11]

Fascia and chronic pain

After reading *A Nation in Pain*, I was struck by the fact that there is not one reference to fascia and its connection to chronic pain. Fascia is the body's seamless web of

---

10 Foreman, Judy. (2014). *A Nation in Pain.* New York, NY: Oxford University Press.
11 Foreman, Judy. (2014). *A Nation in Pain.* New York, NY: Oxford University Press, p. 285.

connective tissue that weaves in and throughout muscles, bones, organs, and cells. As a bodyworker of thirty-plus years who has been treating chronic pain by working with the alignment of the bones and the fascia, I know that fascia is crucial in treating chronic pain, yet it is not spoken about in most medical and academic circles. On my bookshelf sits *Fascia: The Tensional Network of the Human Body,* a 500-page book that covers the science and clinical applications of fascia in manual and movement therapies.[12] Why is this science missing from our discussions on chronic pain?

Those of us working with the fascia do not think of the human body as a skeleton with 206 bones attached together by more than 640 muscles. Western anatomy has been modeled after Newtonian Theory, which breaks things down into parts and ignores the whole. The image of "Muscle Man" fills the anatomical texts used in our medical schools, as well as our schools of massage and alternative medicine, and therefore becomes the dominant way we look at the body. Our bodies are far from being simple robots moving up and down with joints that move our muscles and bones.

What's missing from this picture is the tissue that unites all the parts: the connective tissue, or fascia. Slowly, fascia is becoming more widely known, yet it is still not well understood in many communities. As research into the origin and nature of the fascia comes to the fore, we see that our bodies are seamless webs of connective tissue. Fascia is the only tissue that integrates and forms the support for everything in the body. It is the body's biological fabric. It is the three-dimensional web of fibrous collagen fibers and a gluey gel that holds everything together. In some places it is dense and strong, in others it is highly viscous. The intricate relationship of the fascial system's muscle, bone, ligament, and tendon connections create the perfect balance that unifies and distributes the force of all movement through the body. When one part moves, everything moves. The only tissue that has this kind of responsiveness is the connective tissue. If we use mechanical anatomy, where we analyze the parts, we can destroy the whole and lose continuity with time, space, and the continuum of movement.

---

12 Schleip, Robert, Findley, Thomas W., Chaitow, Leon, and Huijing, Peter A. (2012). *Fascia: The Tensional Network of the Human Body.* Elsevier, Churchill Livingstone.

Holistic Approach

It is time we embrace Einstein's Theory of Relativity and his concepts of space and time not only for all of physics, but for the structural body as well. We are part of a whole system, with subsystems relating to other subsystems within the whole. We should move away from seeing the body as Muscle Man, with our beliefs that muscle and bone are the primary weight-bearing tissues and the primary movers. We can move toward seeing the human body as a dynamic and responsive fascial form, with the possibility of living and moving within the body's harmonious fascial weave the way it was designed. We can embrace this new paradigm for understanding how we are not separate and are actually connected in more ways than we thought.

The importance of a holistic view shows up in our world in more ways than one. The Center for Large Landscape Conservation recently reported that wildlife is at risk for endangerment when cut off from large, connected landscapes in which to live.[13] When we separate our parks and large landscapes from each other by building communities and roads around them, animals lose areas to roam, breed, and nourish themselves with a variety of sustenance. Scientists have noted that species, especially larger ones, have begun dying off as a result. To me, this is a metaphor for the body. When we separate the body into parts, we lose its potential for resiliency and health. The Center for Large Landscape Conservation aims to create a network of connected natural areas resilient to large-scale environmental challenges in an effort to help these species. We need to take the same approach with our bodies. Let us embrace the anatomy of connectivity before we spend billions more on health care with few solutions in treating chronic pain.

---

13 Ament, R., R. Callahan, M. McClure, M. Reuling, and G. Tabor. 2014. Wildlife Connectivity: Fundamentals for conservation action. Center for Large Landscape Conservation: Bozeman, Montana. http://largelandscapes.org/media/publications/Wildlife-Connectivity-Fundamentals-for-Conservation-Action.pdf

CHAPTER 4

DISCOVERING FASCIA

It is a sunny New England day when my new client arrives. After introductions, I ask Steve, who is in his early forties, why he is here. He complains of chronic neck pain he has had for years. His pain mostly occurs on his right side. He has tried massage therapy, physical therapy, and chiropractic, but these methods only helped temporarily.

"My acupuncturist referred me to you," Steve says, "because he thought you might be able to help me with this pain. It gets in the way of my work and it zaps my energy."

His primary care doctor has suggested cortisone shots, and, if that doesn't work, he will refer him for surgery.

"I want to avoid surgery. It makes me nervous thinking about that route of treatment," he adds.

I listen carefully as I take Steve's history. This is where I get clues as to why he might have chronic neck pain. In my paradigm of treatment for pain, it is more important to understand why someone experiences pain rather than what pain they are experiencing.

"Have you had any surgeries or broken bones?" I ask Steve. "Sprained ankles? Any falls in your childhood?" I want to know if any past injuries or strains could be contributing to his pain.

Steve shares that he sprained his right ankle in high school and then again in college while skiing.

"It healed from both sprains," he says, "but I have noticed over the years that my right ankle does not feel as stable as my left ankle."

This history gives me clues to what is happening in Steve's fascial web and where the origin of his neck pain might be. I also ask him what kind of work he does, since this gives me clues as to what kinds of positions his body is in daily.

"I am a graphic designer, and I have created a new software application," he says. "I'm at the computer for hours a day and it's been very stressful lately. I have lots of deadlines." Steve tells me he uses his right hand to click on the mouse and that his hand, particularly his right index finger, has been sore lately.

"What kind of exercise do you do?" I ask Steve. He tells me that even though he spends long hours at the computer, he tries to work out regularly at a gym, runs sporadically, and has begun practicing yoga. He is quite fit, but is still experiencing pain.

"What kind of support systems do you have in your life?" I ask him. Emotional imbalances also show up in the fascia and can contribute to chronic pain patterns. Steve explains that because of his work, he has not had as much time lately for friends and relationships as he would like.

Why do I need to know all of this to understand how I might be able to help Steve with his chronic neck pain? I explain to Steve that my work focuses on treating the fascia, which is the body's only tissue that connects everything together and the only tissue that communicates how we move. This unifying web connects us from head to toe, from skin to bone. Instead of looking at the body as separate muscles and bones, I look at the body as a seamless web of biological fabric that surrounds every muscle, bone, organ, even each individual cell. Since the body and everything in it is connected by this one single biological fabric, it is important to look at where this fabric is pulled, strained, and/or disconnected. Fascia also registers emotional imprints, and therefore healthy fascia is key to our confidence and vibrancy. When our fascial fabric is strained, misaligned, or compressed in any way, the whole fabric responds and our energetic vibrancy is compromised. We often experience chronic pain as a result of this misalignment.

To help Steve understand the importance of fascia and how it might be the missing link to his neck pain, I retrieve a piece of elastic-like fabric from its perch. I envelop Steve's body within the fabric and pull the fabric down at his ankle to show him how that sprained ankle in high school and then again in college might have left an imprint of imbalance in the fascia. We can see the pull in the fabric traveling from Steve's right ankle to the right side of his neck.

"This imbalance in your fascia, which has gone on since high school, may have created a compensation pattern," I explain. "The injury in your fascia didn't stay in your ankle. It traveled throughout the fascial fabric all the way to your neck, because fascia is so interconnected." Steve begins to understand that his neck pain might be related to the fascia in his right ankle.

To help Steve understand this new paradigm of how chronic pain develops, I show him my handheld model of tensegrity. Derived from a basic architectural concept found in nature, a tensegrity structure is one that can hold itself up because of a balance of tensional forces creating suspension and balance. For many years, people thought the body was a continuous *compression* structure, with "the entire body resting like a stack of bricks on the feet."[14] It turns out the body is actually a suspension structure, where bones float in a sea of fascia. In my model, 12-inch wooden rods (representing bones) float suspended by tensional rubber bands (representing fascia). The balance of tensions between the bones and the fascia suspends our joints.

Steve's face lights up: "You mean my body can hold itself up like this structure? I always saw it as weighted down by gravity."

When I push on one side of the tensegrity model, the rods and bands respond and move in different directions. They cluster together at one end and spread out at the other. When I pull instead of push, the rods and bands respond in a different direction. All parts of the system respond to the force. This self-suspending structure stands as a model for how the human body works. To see what a tensegrity structure looks like, turn to Chapter 6.

"Your ankle injury down here," I say as I compress the tensegrity structure at the bottom where Steve's ankle would be, "could be the cause of your neck pain." I show how the structure responds up top where his neck would be. "Often, the symptom is where we feel the pain," I add, "but the cause is somewhere else where we cannot feel the pain. You've been treating the symptom, your neck pain, but we need to find out where the cause is in order to truly relieve it."

I explain to Steve that to treat his chronic pain, we need to look at his body as a whole system connected through a fascial web and suspended through tensegrity. Are his ankle injuries from the past the cause of his neck pain? Have these previous injuries set

---

14 Myers, Thomas. 2014. *Anatomy Trains: Myofascial Meridians for Manual and Movement Therapists, 3rd Edition,* Churchill Livingstone.

up patterns that have disrupted the alignment of his whole fascial web? Where have the major compensation patterns shown up and how have they pulled his body out of alignment? Can we find the original source of the misalignment and remove the cause? How can we restore the alignment so there is balance and ease as well as prevent further injuries and misalignments? Can we prevent the need for cortisone shots or surgery?

These are the questions. Now let's delve into how we might use Steve's brilliant architecture to alleviate his chronic pain.

Chapter 5

Fascia—The Key to Relieving Chronic Pain

In order to unlock the powers of fascia, first we need to understand its properties and its role in our whole-body systems. Fascia, our body-wide fabric, is made up of the strongest fibers in the body (collagen) as well as a gel of gluey proteoglycans, called ground substance. These substances are bathed in a watery medium that, when all is healthy and fluid, communicates a myriad of mechanical functions in the body and has amazing adaptive abilities to all the movements we make. The fascial system enables us to stabilize ourselves, bounce back from stress and strain with resiliency, and move with ease. It has its own sensory nervous system that helps us navigate the forces of gravity and feel our optimal posture. Fascia is our body's spatial medicine. Treating the fascial system is an important avenue into the treatment of chronic pain. Fascia is so crucial because it is one of only three systems that hold our body's complete shape and, therefore, has a major influence in our whole-body health.

What Shape Are You In?

I'm not asking if you have gone to the gym or worked out lately. What I want to know is how does your body shape itself? What shapes your body's design and architecture? What are the containers and shapes within your architecture and why are you shaped this way?

The largest single organ in the body is the skin, which shows us our shape. Yet, the skin just shows us the outer surface of the body, and we are not able to see the body's complex, inner dimensions. If everything in your body under the skin was visible, you would see three anatomical systems that show the exact shape of your body: the nervous system, the circulatory system, and the fascial system.[15] These systems are all fluid systems. For a moment, let's look at them separately, even though they are never separate nor ever function without each other.

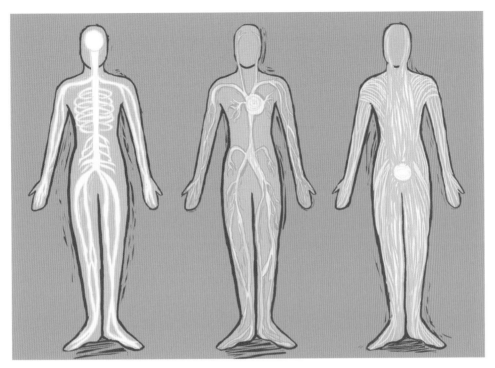

The body's three nets that show our shape: the neural net, with the brain at its center (left); the circulatory net, with the heart at its center (middle); and the fascial net, with the body's center of gravity at its center (right).

The neural net

If we took all other systems out of the body, we could see the complex neural network that lives within us. I saw an example of the neural net at the Body Worlds Exhibit when it first came to Boston in 2007. Each Body Worlds exhibition contained real human specimens, including whole-body plastinates, as well as individual organs and transparent body slices.[16] Looking at the representations of the neural net, I could see the brain, the

---

15 Myers, Thomas. 2014. *Anatomy Trains: Myofascial Meridians for Manual and Movement Therapists, 3rd Edition,* Churchill Livingstone, p. 32.

16 See more about Body Worlds at http://www.bodyworlds.com/en.html

spinal cord, and all the nerves branching out to each part of the body; in sum, they created the shape of the entire human body!

When the nervous system is working well, it is communicating to all parts of the body. It produces coordinated, fast responses to internal and external stimulation. Your body depends on the rapid-fire nerve endings of the nervous system to signal that you need to pull your hand away from the fire or step out of the way of that speeding car. This system communicates through neural tube-like structures that carry encoded information, usually in an on–off form. The physiological center is the brain, the largest and densest plexus of neurons.

The circulatory net

The vascular system also shows us the exact shape of the human body. The center of this fluid system is the heart, which pumps blood to and from the lungs out to all the arteries, even out to those tiny capillaries, and receives blood back from the veins. An exhibit at Body Worlds showed this fluid system extracted from the body. To see the shape of the body with only its veins and arteries right down to those tiny capillaries is a sight to behold. Mesmerizing!

The circulatory net communicates chemical information around the body in the fluid blood using cylindrical structures called capillaries that feed every nook and cranny within. This net communicates more slowly than the neural net. This is why it takes about twenty minutes before your pain medication reaches the area of pain.

The fascial net

The third whole-body communicating network that shows our shape is the fascial system. Until recently, we had not paid much attention to this system and its importance. This system shows us the whole body, inside and out. If we were to look at just the fascial system, the outer layer would take the shape of our body like a leotard; it is called the superficial layer and resides just under our skin, like the backing of a carpet. This layer wraps around, connects with, and intertwines down in and around all the muscles, bones, and organs. We would see the thick parts in ligaments, tendons, cartilage, and bones, especially around the joints. We would see our muscles, muscle cells, and bundles of cells encased in it and infused with it like a cotton candy net. Organs, such as the heart, liver, pancreas, and brain, are contained in fascial sacs. No part of our body is separate from this net, head to toe, skin to bone. This three-dimensional net is linked together through the ligaments, bones, tendons, and muscles. The fascial web permeates the body in such an intricate way that it even supports every cell! Without the fascial net to contain us, our muscles and bones would fall to the ground in a heap, our brain would be uncongealed, and our organs would spill out into the abdominal cavity. We cannot take out anything from the body without bringing some of this ubiquitous fascial tissue with us. In addition, the fascial net is also the scaffolding for the neural and circulatory nets, as well as the lymph system.

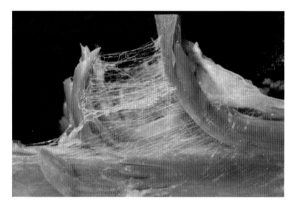

Fascia, the body's biological fabric. Reproduced with kind permission from Ronald Thompson.

Dr. Jean-Claude Guimberteau, a French surgeon, was the first person to use endoscopy to reveal living fascia, our first view into this unique imagery of living fascia at work in the living body. Thanks to his research, we can now see the gluey, elastic, responsive, and dynamic interplay of this body-wide system, which he calls the *sliding system,* and its ability to adapt and self-organize in ways we never knew before.[17] I could not believe my eyes when I viewed Dr. Guimberteau's video at the First International Fascia Research Congress in Boston in 2007. As a result of his work, my ideas have changed, the way I look at the body has changed, and my touch has changed. I can never again see the body as a set of separate bones, ligaments, tendons, and muscles. Instead, I now view the body as a seamless web of connection that holds the fluid dynamics of inner communication. What Dr. Guimberteau has done is shift the

17 Guimberteau, Jean-Claude. 2015. *Architecture of Human Living Fascia.* Edinburgh: Handspring Publishing.

paradigm of how the body works from the inside out. Through Dr. Guimberteau's images in his videos and his most recent book, *Architecture of Human Living Fascia* (2015), we can now actually see a body-wide continuity in a way we have never seen before. We will look back at our old model of Muscle Man and see it as outdated. I am delighted to share with you now this new anatomy of the future. I love to show my clients and colleagues these photographs and videos. A picture is worth a thousand words, and in this case that statement is so true.

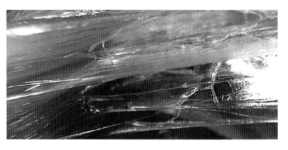

Unfortunately, the fascial net has been ignored by most artists, scientists, researchers, and the medical world. Western anatomy tended to ignore this all-encompassing net—except the parts that are easy to see: the ligaments, tendons, cartilage, and bones—

Photo of living fascia intertwining and interweaving with muscle fibers. Reproduced with kind permission from Jean-Claude Guimberteau.

thinking it was just packing material. It was often discarded in medical school dissections. Yet if we look more closely at fascia, especially living fascia, we see its mucus-like structure filled with bound water. We can then more fully understand fascia's role in connecting, hydrating, and nourishing every single part of the body. Could it be that because X-rays, MRIs, CAT scans, or electromyography are not looking at fascia, we are missing one of the links to treating chronic pain?

Due to the wealth of new science on fascia coming from the world of bodyworkers turned scientists, we are starting to figure out some of the reasons for chronic pain. This research is not coming out of the medical or academic circles. It is coming out of the circles of bodyworkers who want to understand their own work more deeply. Scientists often dismissed bodyworkers, but are now beginning to pay attention to what is unfolding. We are just beginning to see and to understand that the fascia could be the most important tissue in the body to help us address the issue of chronic pain. And it is this tissue that has the necessary architecture to hold us all together, to align us, to balance us, to center us, to keep us vibrant and healthy.

Fascia: Our Resilient Spiderweb

The fascial net communicates through tube-like structures, but they are not the same construction as the tubes in the neural and circulatory nets. The basic unit of the fascial net is a collagen fibril, which is a cell product. A collagen fibril is more like a three-strand rope. This is what makes fascia strong. We can use the image of a collagen tube that is long and cable-like.[18] These collagen cables communicate mechanical information. For example, what is happening at a joint when we are lifting a weight or dancing the tango and the intricate balance between tension and compression is being conveyed through the fascial net. In addition, the crushing pressure of stuck, misaligned fascia on muscles, nerves, blood vessels, and bones is also being conveyed through this tissue. It just may be where chronic inflammation resides. (Do not get this mixed up with the stretch receptors that live in the muscles, like muscle spindles and Golgi tendon organs, which signal to the nervous system in its usual encoded way about what is happening in the myofascial net.) The fascial net communicates in a unique way. It communicates through simple pulls and pushes along lines and sheaths of the fabric, from fiber to fiber, cell to cell. A tug in the fascial net is communicated across the entire system. Tug on the thread of your sweater and the whole sweater responds. Tug on the thread of a spiderweb and the whole web responds.

I like the analogy of a spiderweb with its sticky, gluey threads woven into a specific design. A spider weaves its web using its ancient instincts into an intricate design. An insect flies into the web and gets stuck. The weight of the insect pulls on the threads of the web and changes the shape of the web. The web reacts with the forces of gravity. The spider comes in and uses her "hands" to gently remove the insect from the web. The web springs back to its original shape quite easily. It is resilient, like our fascial net. "Insects" fly into our web: we get an injury playing a sport or have an accident, we undergo surgery, we experience emotional events in our childhood. Unfortunately, we do not always have the wise hands of a spider (hands-on practitioner) to come in and remove the imprint from our web. The imprint remains in the web, and compensation patterns occur as our

---

18 Myers, Thomas. 2014. *Anatomy Trains: Myofascial Meridians for Manual and Movement Therapists, 3rd Edition*, Churchill Livingstone, p. 32.

web negotiates the imbalances and the pull of gravity on us. We are usually not aware that our web is making these adjustments because they are happening on such microscopic levels, especially at important structures like our foundation and semi-foundation joints.

Most injuries occur in the fascia—especially in the ligaments and tendons at joint structures—not in the muscles. The fascial adjustments can happen very slowly and over days, months, and years, or they can happen quickly. Our web changes its shape around the original imprint. The fascia gets stuck and dehydrated. The fluidity our fascia needs to communicate gets thwarted. As our body compensates for the imprint and the effects of gravity, the web becomes less balanced and, thus, vulnerable. We might experience another injury on top of the original one, have unexpected surgery, or experience another traumatic emotional event that weakens it further. We feel soreness, achiness, or stiffness. Low-level inflammation builds. Our fascia responds to the stress and strain by laying down more bone and more fascia. A bone spur can develop as a strained ligament gets sheared. Our spine starts torqueing into side curves as we tend to sink into one hip while we stand (scoliosis). Or, too much compression in one part of the spine puts stress on another part (kyphosis or hunch back). All these events and imprints start to change our fascial shape. Our alignment, our posture, our breathing, our moods, our resiliency or ability to bounce back from physical and emotional impacts are all affected.

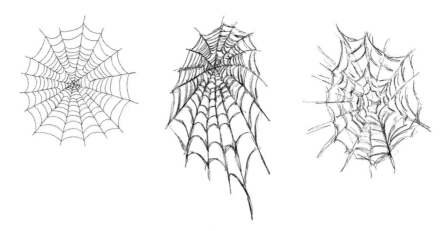

Spiderweb aligned, pulled out of alignment, and dehydrated after chronic misalignment.

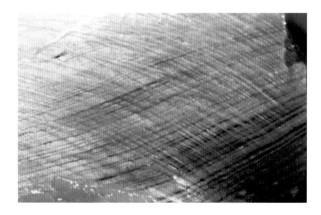

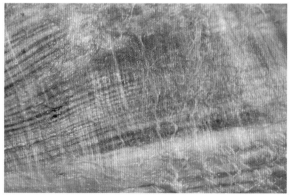

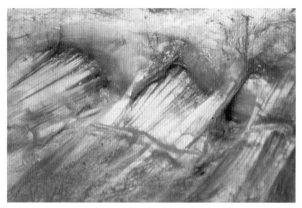

Photos of healthy fascia (top left), strained fascia (top right), and hardened fascia (bottom left). Reproduced with kind permission from Ronald Thompson.

Fascia Holds Our Physical and Emotional Imprints

As a practitioner who has been working in the body for many years, it is my job to discover where the clients' imprints reside in the fascial net and the compensation patterns that have evolved from those imprints. This is why I take an extensive history when I first meet a client. First, I ask what the issue of pain is. Then I ask about past injuries, surgeries, accidents, falls, and their line of work. Ideally, I want to find the original imprint into the fascial web.

When I ask my clients what support systems they have, the answers give me a sense of how the challenges, struggles, and issues with family, friends, and partners may have affected the fascial web. Emotional imprints are as important as physical imprints. Since fascia is the communicator of mechanical and emotional issues (which have mechanical impact), it is important to also understand emotional imprints. As a practitioner, I want to understand the person's patterns of compensation so I can support him/her in moving them out of the web. It is my job to find where the first imprint threw the fascial net out of balance. If I can use my hands to remove the original imprint (read more about this in Chapter 7), my hope is that we can remove the pulls and strains, which, in turn, relieves the symptoms showing up as chronic pain in the web. Once the fascial web is realigned, we use subtle movement to sustain that alignment (more on this in Parts 3 and 4).

Body-mind connection

Those of us working on the body believe that the body and mind are inseparable. It no longer works to say the mind and memory are located only in the brain. Systems of hands-on therapy have documented that a portion of memory is "body memory," or "tissue-held memory." Memory, emotion, and experiences, especially traumatic events in childhood, are stored in the body as vibrational imprints in our tissues. These imprints can keep a memory, emotion, or event stuck in our behavior. (Read more about this in Chapters 10 and 11.)

Dr. Fritz Smith, the creator of Zero Balancing, has a theory that the location of the tissue-held memory is partially based on how we received the original information. Dr. Smith believes that the soft tissues, muscles, ligaments, and organs have the ability to react when an imprint comes into our web. They can expand, contract, or in some way interact with the imprint. He believes that imprints on reactive tissue or an organ will be held closer to consciousness than with nonreactive tissue. Bone, periosteum (the fascial envelope around all bones), and cartilage are nonreactive tissues. Since they don't have the ability to react, all they can do is receive imprints. These imprints bury deeply into the bone layer of the web. Bones are where our deep core issues are held. Our early childhood losses often go into bone, our issues of identity, sense of purpose, our stance in the world, our sense of personal security.[19]

---

19 Smith, Fritz Frederick, MD. (2005). *Alchemy of Touch Moving Through Mastery Through the Lens of Zero Balancing.* Taos, NM: Complementary Medicine Press.

Bodywork in the Fascia

Whether we hold imprints in the deeper layer of fascia, in the bone, or in the soft tissue layers, removing the imprint, whichever layer it is in, may be helpful in assisting the fascial web to rebalance, realign, and restore its health and relieve pain. One way to remove a fascial imprint is through hands-on therapy or bodywork that focuses on the fascia. In the world of complementary medicine, certain modalities treat specific layers of the fascia. Some of these modalities are Fascial Release Technique, Myofascial Release Technique, Rolfing, and Structural Integration. Certain modalities treat the superficial fascia closer to the skin and around the muscles. Other modalities, such as Osteopathy and Zero Balancing, treat the deeper layers closer to the bones and joints. Some modalities even treat the dura mater, the tough outermost membrane enveloping the brain and spinal cord.

To release the fascia, a skilled hands-on therapist or bodyworker may use several conscious touch techniques. One way is a direct approach in which the practitioner sinks down into the layers of tissue using finely tuned trained hands until a layer of resistance is felt. This is where the fascia is stuck. Once there, the practitioner waits until that resistance releases. By being aware of the layers and molding her hand to the shape of the body part being worked, she causes the fascial tissue to release, the fibers to lengthen, and the gelatin-like ground substance to change from hard and stuck to soft and pliable. The practitioner uses her second hand to hold length, width, and space as the tissues release. Another way to release fascia is using an indirect approach. With this approach the dysfunctional, tight, and held tissues are guided along the path of least resistance until the tissue relaxes and free movement is achieved.

It is important that the practitioner be sensitive enough to know which layer to work and not to push past the layer of resistance. If a practitioner pushes past this resistance, the client will experience pain and his body will reject the message of release from the practitioner's touch. Over time, as the layers release, the body learns a rich vocabulary of touch, and the communication between the practitioner and the client deepens.

Note: *Whatever you learn in this book will be enhanced by working with a skilled hands-on practitioner in bodywork or movement to assist you in releasing stuck fascia so that chronic pain, poor posture, and dysfunctional movement habits can be addressed. You can then engage in a new training of your fascial net that will allow you to sustain whole-body alignment. The movement training in Part 4, while effective on its own, will be greatly enhanced by hands-on bodywork. I highly recommend seeking out a practitioner to accompany you on this journey to relieving your chronic pain.*

Sustainable Bodywork

There is an array of hands-on therapy or bodywork practitioners and movement educators available today who have excellent methods for dealing with chronic pain. Personally, I have explored many of these techniques and worked with highly skilled practitioners and movement teachers who have been immensely helpful in my journey into a healthy, vibrant, and pain-free life. I am indebted to their wisdom and support.

Often what was missing for me in my experience after certain fascial release sessions was that only certain areas of my body were being treated. Because of my experience with Zero Balancing, I yearned to be touched as a whole and experience whole-body alignment and healing. In other hands-on bodywork sessions, even when I would feel like I was touched as a whole body and aligned beautifully, I could not sustain that release and feeling of alignment when I went about everyday life. I yearned for a way to be touched and aligned as a whole body *and* a way to sustain that feeling of wholeness and alignment on a day-to-day basis.

As a hands-on therapist, I focus on deep inner core alignment in each session. Other modalities focus on the body in its separate parts and integrate them as a final step. When I work with the body, I connect and integrate the whole fascial web and skeleton in each session. I want my clients to feel integration from the beginning and throughout the session. Instead of analyzing the parts of the body and telling my clients what is out of alignment, I focus on what is in alignment and how the body is designed brilliantly. This is what makes Sustainable Body different; it addresses the whole dynamic system that you are. It also teaches you how to sustain that alignment on your own at home.

From my many years of experience—having my layers of fascia released and releasing those layers in my clients, having the bones and ligaments of my foundation and semi-foundation joints balanced and aligned as a whole and doing the same for my clients, and learning to move and align myself from the deeper layers of my core and to teach that to my clients—I grew Sustainable Body training. I found that by going deep into the inner core layers of the body at the level of bone and the deeper layers of fascia, I could feel alignment, balance, strength, and flexibility more directly, and I could sustain it. And, I could teach others to do the same!

This is what makes Sustainable Body training different from many other methods you may have tried. If you can align the inner core of your whole body once a day, you are more likely to be aligned and balanced and thus free of chronic pain.

Fascia Is the Key

We now understand that the fascial net holds our shape and connects every part of the body from head to toe, skin to bone. Fascia is how the body holds itself up and is the root of our posture. Fascia is the scaffolding for the neural, circulatory, and lymph systems. In addition, fascia is the tissue that registers our imprints from injuries, surgeries, and life. The good news is that fascia can be remodeled back to its original shape. Using the hands of a skilled practitioner or movements designed to create space in the tissues and joints, fascia can be melted, realigned, and rehydrated. (Read more about how this happens in Chapter 7.) It is through the fascia that we can reclaim our "kid body" (the natural way we used to move as children) and live a pain-free life regardless of age, culture, race, body type, or level of activity.

CHAPTER 6

TENSEGRITY

Unlike the spiderweb, which relies on an external framework for support, the body is a self-contained unit that supports itself. How does the body hold itself up? To understand how our musculoskeletal system's brilliant architecture works, it is helpful to understand the concept of tensegrity. Tensegrity is a term for tensional integrity, or floating compression. Tensegrity forms are self-stabilized, independent of gravity, and need no external support.

Based on the discovery by artist Kenneth Snelson and coined by the visionary and genius Buckminster Fuller (1895–1983), tensegrity is a basic architectural concept. It describes a structural relationship principle that Fuller defined as stabilizing the shape of structures by continuous tension, rather than continuous compression.[20] Continuous compression forces are used to hold up a stone arch or a tall building. Yet it is possible to design structures where a continuous tension network—the integrity of tensions, hence tensegrity—can suspend floating, firm rods that do not touch one another, but are suspended and made strong by the network of balanced compression and tensile parts. In other words, when two sets of forces—the compression force and the tension force—are balanced, suspension is created. The resulting forms are lightweight, resilient, and can withstand dynamic stress by distributing a load to all parts of the structure simultaneously. These structures are able to yield under increasing loads without breaking or coming apart. Prior to the mid-twentieth century, the principle of tensegrity was unknown. It is an important discovery of our time.[21]

---

20 Fuller, Buckminster as referenced in: Myers, Thomas. 2014. *Anatomy Trains: Myofascial Meridians for Manual and Movement Therapists, 3rd Edition,* Churchill Livingstone. pp. 44–50.
21 Scarr, Graham. 2014. *Biotensegrity: The Structural Basis of Life*. Handspring Publishing, pp.1–10.

Architects have been using the principle of tensegrity to design buildings, and engineers and scientists have been using the principle in all sorts of design, from satellites and robots to furniture and toys. For many decades now a few scientists have been applying the concept to living structures by exploring the links between tensegrity and biological structures. When scientists observed biological organisms, from the smallest to the largest, they found that all biological organisms are made strong and resilient by their balance of tension and compression forces.

Biotensegrity

One of these pioneers, orthopedic and spine surgeon Dr. Stephen Levin, originated the concept of biotensegrity more than thirty years ago.[22] Levin noticed that when he tightened up the cruciate ligaments during knee joint surgery, the bones moved apart. This did not fall into the old anatomy of the joints as lever systems. He also noticed that "normal joints always had a slight spacing between the bones" and that there was no way to explain this space.[23] This led him to see the tensegrity of the body, its biotensegrity. It was like the bones were "floating" in the soft tissues.[24] Dr. Levin's influence on others in the fields of medicine and bodywork continues.

Our tensegrity architecture provides a continuous network of restricting but adjustable tension. The old model of Newtonian mechanics of levers and hinges, which was first described by a mathematician in 1680, no longer applies to our fascial bodies. Our skeletal system is part of the biotensegritous matrix. Our bones—also connective tissue—form the struts of stable compression for a large part of the body's structure. The fascia provides the tensile pull in a continuous sea of balanced elastic members. They do not touch each other. Bones are like spacers that float within the fascial network. The tone and fluidity of the fascial fabric determines a balanced body and the suspension in the joints. The continuity of the fascial system does not end at the bones and joints; it

---

22 Levin, Stephen M. 2016. http://biotensegrity.com/
23 Stephen M. Levin as cited in: Scarr, Graham. 2014. *Biotensegrity: The Structural Basis of Life*. Handspring Publishing, 61.
24 Stephen M. Levin as cited in: Scarr, Graham. 2014. *Biotensegrity: The Structural Basis of Life*. Handspring Publishing, 61.

contains and incorporates muscles, bones, joints, and organs. It is managing and integrating all movement with resilience and strength. Bodyworkers have also been inspired to use tensegrity as a model for how the human structure holds itself in balanced suspension. Our bodies are layer upon layer of tensegrity structure and function. Tensegrity structures are efficient and adaptive and may help us understand how connected our musculoskeletal system is in new and important ways.

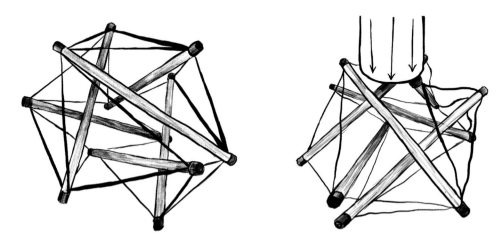

A tensegrity structure when balanced and suspended (left) and responding to an external imprint (right).

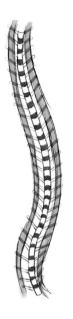

If we look at the spine as a biotensegrity structure, we can see that the natural curves and fluidity are designed to absorb and distribute tensional forces and shock in every movement we make.

It makes sense that our bodies evolved over time, creating our biotensegrity structures as ways to be structurally balanced and also highly adaptive to the various movements we need to make. This architectural design offers maximum strength for bones, fascia, and muscles to all work together. Yet the stability of the tensegrity structure is not stiff and rigid, it is resilient and buoyant because of the continuous movement of forces within the fascial web.

Keep in mind that our biotensegrity bodies are designed so well that:

1. A minimal amount of energy is used to maintain its shape because it is stable in all directions. This is why alignment of the bones, muscles, and fascia is so important!

2. Strain in one part of the body affects everything else because our structure absorbs force throughout all the elements in it. Strain created from a sprained ankle or the impact of surgery affects alignment throughout the whole body.

3. Tension in one part of the body is distributed throughout the body. Tension and misalignment of one joint, especially a foundation or semi-foundation joint, is felt everywhere in the body and you may not even realize it.

4. Because our tensegrity structure can manage tension and distribute strain evenly, it responds to alignment and misalignment as a whole system. Therefore, we need to treat the body as a whole and not just the parts.

5. The weakest link in the structure is where the symptom of pain occurs, not necessarily the cause of the pain. To relieve chronic pain, we need to address the cause and not just treat the symptom.

6. The entire system, the whole body, must be freed to restore alignment and suspension.

Chronic pain needs to be addressed with a whole-systems approach.

Tensegrity at the Cellular Level

Donald E. Ingber, MD, PhD,[25] was the first to recognize that tensegrity architecture is a fundamental principle that governs how living cells are structured to respond

---

25 Founding Director and Core Faculty, Wyss Institute at Harvard University, Professor of Vascular Biology at Harvard Medical School and Vascular Biology Program, Boston Children's Hospital

biochemically to mechanical forces. Cells themselves are tensegrity structures in which each cell contains a balance of tension and compression elements. Cells are microcosms of the body with self-supporting functions that, in turn, support all larger biological functions. The cell's compression struts are called the cytoskeleton. The cytoskeleton weaves through the cell's interior as strands of filament and microtubules. These microtubules provide a communication system within the cell and flow with fluid. His work in mechanobiology shed light on the fact that the cytoskeleton is an important part of the communication system within the cell. Studies of how the body's physical forces and mechanics impact development, health prevention, and treatment of diseases are just being explored. Dr. Ingber's study proposes that mechanics-driven or direct physical stimulation could one day replace or enhance drug-based treatments for pain. What this boils down to is that manual or hands-on therapy is found to remodel the fascial matrix, or tensegrity, of the cells, which helps create a more optimal environment for the cells and eventually allows a restoration of balance within the body.[26]

Thanks to the intellectual fortitude of many who stepped out of the box and did the research, we are able to understand and apply the concepts of tensegrity to the body, biotensegrity, in new and important ways. Using this concept, we can understand more clearly how the body has a global response to a local mechanical stress. We see how the body has a network to deal with the mechanical demands imposed on it, while at the same time ensures an absorption of the forces we deal with every day. We see how the body maintains equilibrium and space. We can see how this balance is seen even at the cellular level and could have profound influences on our cellular health. By viewing the body with its fascinating network of balance between tension and compression among bones and fluid fascia, we can approach chronic pain from a new perspective.

---

26 Ingber, Donald. 1998 Jan. The Architecture of Life. *Scientific American; 278:* 48–57. Retrieved from http://time.arts.ucla.edu/Talks/Barcelona/Arch_Life.htm For more information, you can visit the following websites: http://wyss.harvard.edu/viewpage/121/donald-e-ingber and www.childrenshospital.org/research/ingber

CHAPTER 7

THE NEUROFASCIAL SYSTEM

In the 1980s, a dispute arose in the bodywork community between practitioners of the Feldenkrais Method of somatic education (movement) and practitioners of the Rolfing Method of Structural Integration (fascia). Feldenkrais practitioners believed that chronic pain came from restrictions in the body stemming from neuromuscular signals in the brain, and Rolfing practitioners believed that chronic pain came from restrictions in the body stemming from stuck fascia. To find out which group was correct, an experiment was performed. It was observed that muscle restrictions disappeared during general anesthesia. What was going on? Was it the fascial system or the nervous system that carried the body's pain signals?

The bodyworkers-turned-scientists delved into this question, which led fascial scientists to study the mechano-sensory nature of fascia and its ability to respond to hands-on therapy. Their research led to a rethinking of traditional hands-on therapies and to the first neurologically oriented model of the effects of fascial manipulation. There was a lot more happening in the fascia than we ever realized. The sensory nerves within the fascia were more varied and ubiquitous than suspected. Because of the sensory capacity of fascia, it is the fascia that serves as a body-wide mechanosensitive signaling system, with a function like the nervous system, yet separate and unique in its abilities. These discoveries led to a deeper understanding and, thus, to a new perspective of the body: the neurofascial system.

Fascia plays a major role in whole body communication. It is our richest sensory organ. Unlike muscle, the fascia does not receive input from the brain or the nervous system. There are no motor nerves in fascia. Instead, there is a wealth of sensory nerves in fascia. Fascia has ten times more sensory nerve endings than in muscle tissue.[27] The latest studies show there is a massive amount of communication occurring within the body with little input from the central nervous system or the brain. Cell to cell, organ to organ, joint to joint communication is occurring on an electrical and vibrational level through the fluid system of the fascia. More signals come through the connective tissue than through the nervous system.

Fascia Has Its Own Nervous System

The neurofascial system has its own ways of communicating separate from the central nervous system and the brain. This communication comes from different kinds of sensory nerves. Sensory receptors, called proprioceptors and mechanoreceptors, sense position and movement within the body and are triggered by misalignment, squeezing, stretching, and compression. They sense pressure or the sudden shift in a joint, an impact to the body, and the pulls and strains in the fascial web. These sensory nerves give us the ability to sense where our body is in relation to gravity as well as in relation to the space around us.

The mechanical information being communicated throughout our fascial web occurs in two ways, or in two rhythms: one rapid and one slow. The interplay of tension and compression being communicated travels at the speed of sound, more quickly than the nervous system. This information is taken in and transmitted through sensory receptors that live in the fascia.

Sometimes, the mechanical information is transmitted at a slower rate, and it may take days, weeks, or even years for this information to be communicated. As a manual therapist, I often find, through conscious touch (see below), that an injury or surgery from many years ago ends up as chronic pain in a place in the body that's far from the original imprint. When there is chronic misalignment over time, these sensory nerves alert the brain to potential damage. Low-level inflammation builds without your conscious awareness. Every slight motion and its nuances of changing mechanical

---

27 Myers, Thomas. (2011, Mar 23). Fascial Fitness: Training in the NeuroMyofascial Web. *IDEA Fitness Journal, 8*(4). Retrieved from http://www.ideafit.com/fitness-library/fascial-fitness

forces is noticed by the sensory receptors in your fascial net. The crushing pressure on the bones, joints, and muscles is registered through your sensory nerves. If the pressure, strain, or pull is not addressed, your fascia gets stuck. These stuck, nonmoving places are called fascial adhesions. Without movement, fascia dehydrates. In addition, the signaling through the fascial fluids diminishes. Your fascia cannot communicate well, and you lose your ability to move fluidly and to connect to your stability.

How the neurofascial system communicates

A more recent discovery is that the sensory nerves in your fascia do not need the central nervous system to communicate with each other. This body-wide communication system depends on the unique qualities and properties of the fascia. Connective tissue is made up of strong collagen fibers embedded in a gel-like ground substance. It is seen that the fibers are arranged in highly ordered crystalline arrangements. Like other crystals, connective tissue is piezoelectric, which means it generates electric fields when it is compressed or stretched. This ability to conduct an electrodynamic field is due to the liquid crystalline collagen fibers of the connective tissues. Any movement of any part in the body generates electrical fields that spread through the surrounding tissues. Since collagen is a semiconductor, connective tissue is comparable to an integrated electronic network that allows every single part of the body to communicate with each other. This interconnected electronic fabric that is elastic, flexible, strong, and resilient depends on the continuous flow of information through its sliding, gliding, hydrated fabric.[28]

The speed of communication in this system is much faster than what we know of nerve conduction. We might think of these non-neural cells in the fascia as tiny crystalline ears that are listening to the constant stream of messages radiating out from nerves and muscles. They use this information to adjust their activities. Scientists have also documented that the particles in the fascia move in a wave-like pattern, which enables the information to spread rapidly throughout the body. These liquid crystals make rapid

---

28 Oschman, James L., Ph.D. *Readings on the Scientific Basis of Bodywork and Movement Therapies.* www. somatics.de

changes and respond to electric and magnetic fields. They also respond to changes in temperature, pressure, shear forces, and hydration.[29]

Many of these proprioceptive nerves, which are designed to sense position and movement, reside in large concentrations at joint junctures where muscles, bones, ligaments, tendons, and cartilage intersect.

Ligaments communicate too

Another discovery the fascial scientists made is that there is a wealth of communication occurring in our ligaments, in the bone, and in the fascial wrapping around the bone (periosteum). In the old anatomy, ligaments were separate from bone and were there to connect bone to bone and to be used for mechanical movement. In the new anatomy, these richly innervated tissues play a key role in sensory perception. These receptors are designed to communicate signals in the body between the autonomic nervous system and the fascial system. In areas where the fascia is more dense—for example, in joints that allow for little dislocation or deformation, such as the low back and the arches of the feet—these ligaments have receptors that are designed to cope with the functional architecture in the joints. They are sensitive to deformation in a joint, but this signal is under our conscious awareness. Because of this unique architecture and sensory perception, fascial scientists have given these ligaments a new name: dynamic ligaments, or "dynaments." Dynaments are an architectural unit the body uses to communicate between bone and fascia and relay some of the deepest signals in the body. These are the architectural units that connect our biotensegrity structure so the bones can float in a sea of elastic fascia effortlessly.

Before the brain signals the muscles to move, the fascia prepares the body by creating tensegrity to minimize friction and compression in the joints, where many of these dynaments or ligaments reside. In order to align and stabilize joints, fascia creates what is called "pre-anticipatory tensional stress" between the joints. This body-wide

---

29 Ho, Mae-Wan, and White, David P. The Acupuncture System and The Liquid Crystalline Collagen Fibers of the Connective Tissues. American Journal of Complementary Medicine (in press). Institute of Science in Society www.i-sis.org.uk/lcm.php.

prestressing lets the brain know how much motor nerve impulse to send to muscles to create proper leverage, contraction, and timing. This supportive tension allows the body to remain balanced as we perform our movements. It is my hypothesis that much of this supportive tension comes through the deep fascial inner Vertical Core and its center of gravity, where the slow-twitch fibers of this core communicate—more on this in Chapters 9 and 10.

The Interoceptive Nerves—A New Way of Communicating

New research shows that there are two kinds of sensory nerves in fascia. The ones that register mechanical information (as discussed previously), like the misalignment in a joint, are myelinated, or encapsulated, nerve endings. There is another group of sensory receptors that are unmyelinated, or unencapsulated, nerve endings. Scientists call them free nerve endings, and they have opened up a new field in fascial research: interoception.[30] These nerve endings register the balance and homeostasis in the body's internal spaces, like the organs, and in important joint structures that create stability and balance. They fire into a deeper part of the brain (anterior cortex) and are registering what our subconscious is sensing in our body.

Research presented at the International Fascia Research Congress (Abstracts 2007, 2009, 2012) documents that these sensory nerve fibers, called interstitial myofascial tissue receptors, are abundant in fascia and are hardly mentioned in most textbooks. Is it possible that these sensory nerves are the link into our autonomic nervous system, the system responsible for the involuntary actions of our internal organs, such as breathing and digesting?

With the fascial system of interoception, which is sensing homeostasis within the body, we may be able to better understand how fascia is intimately linked to the peripheral nervous system, which is located outside the brain and spinal cord (central nervous

---

30 Schleip, Robert, Findley, Thomas W., Chaitow, Leon, and Huijing, Peter A. (2012). *Fascia The Tensional Network of the Human Body,* Churchill Livingstone. p. 89–94.

system).[31] The peripheral nervous system resides in the outer parts of the body and is connected through our fascial fabric.

The peripheral nervous system includes the autonomic nervous system, which is responsible for regulation of internal organs and glands, and it controls our involuntary actions including breathing, digestion, organ functions, etc. All involuntary functions in the body are regulated by the autonomic nervous system, which consists of three subsystems:

1. Sympathetic nervous system: activates our stress response, commonly known as the fight-or-flight response.
2. Parasympathetic nervous system: stimulates the relaxation response, commonly known as the rest-and-digest response. (Note: The parasympathetic nervous system registers the freeze response, see Chapter 11.)
3. Enteric nervous system: controls the gastrointestinal system, organ-to-organ communication.

Because of the intimate connection between the autonomic nervous system and the fascia, we may be able to balance and regulate these systems by treating the fascial system directly. If regulation is out of balance due to stress or not enough rest, our vital functions go into overdrive. Energy goes into monitoring vital functions, like the heart, liver, and kidneys. As a result, other functions, like hair growth and muscle repair, get less energy. This imbalance accelerates aging and depresses repair of all tissues and the immune system. This imbalance is likely a precursor to chronic pain.

The relationship between the autonomic nervous system and the fascial system is more important than we realized. Because of the almost instantaneous communication occurring within the interoceptive system of fascia, when the autonomic nervous system is imbalanced, the fascial system is imbalanced, and vice versa. It does not matter which comes first—stuck fascia or an imbalanced autonomic nervous system—they are intimately linked. They are always influencing each other. You could be physically fit, but

---

31 Staugaard-Jones, JoAnn. (2012.) *The Vital Psoas Muscle Connecting Physical, Emotional, and Spiritual Well-Being. Berkeley, CA: North Atlantic Books.* pp.75–76.

your breathing may be shallow or your digestive tract tight. Whether you have a healthy or unhealthy lifestyle, an active or inactive one, the balance between these systems determines your health and your response to chronic pain. (Conscious touch, gentle stretching, and breathing softly, slowly and deeply is what balances these systems. See Chapters 9 and 13.)

New research shows us what we did not know until now: we can rebalance the autonomic nervous system and the fascial system (the neurofascial system) together. The cause of chronic pain could be the stuck stress of life or poor posture, repetitive movements, gut disorders, poor body-wide communication, dehydrated and inflamed fascia, misaligned joints, anxiety, or depression. The autonomic nervous system needs the fascial system to be fluid and hydrated for communication of homeostasis.

Conscious Touch of the Neurofascial System

There are two ways to rehydrate and rebalance the neurofascial system: through conscious touch and through conscious movement. Here I describe how a skilled practitioner may use conscious touch and conscious movement as a way to treat the neurofascial system, and thus rebalance the whole body using this system.

How to touch the neurofascia

Earlier, you learned that fascia holds your imprints, which can be held at various layers of the fascia, and that a skilled hands-on practitioner may use one or several conscious touch techniques to release fascia. (See Bodywork in the fascia in Chapter 5.) Delving deeper into this subject, it is interesting to note that touching connective tissue, or fascia, takes different training and skills than working with muscles, as is done in massage. This is because fascia has different qualities than muscle. Muscle tissue is composed of fibers capable of shortening or lengthening to move a body part. Muscle tissue is elastic and has its own blood supply.

Touching or massaging a muscle allows it to relax and rest, yet the muscle remains at a certain resting length and width. The relaxation effects felt in muscles are often temporary, especially if there is stuck stress in the fascia around those muscles, and/or around the organs of the autonomic nervous system. Since fascia envelops and weaves throughout your muscles, connects muscles to bone, connects bone to bone, and envelops each organ, it needs to be treated as well. Yet, fascia needs to be touched in a slightly different way than muscle.

As you learned, fascia is our richest sensory organ, with numerous sensory nerve endings that are communicating to each and every part of the body. Because of the unique qualities of fascia—collagen fibers and a matrix of ground substance that is malleable and bathed in lots of bound water—when it is touched in a skilled and conscious way, fascia melts into a pliable and more liquid-like state. When in this more pliable state, the ability of your body to communicate through its fascial fluids increases, and balance and ease are accessed.

The skillful therapist uses conscious touch and gentle traction or stretching to stimulate the two kinds of sensory nerves in the fascia: the myelinated nerve endings, the ones that register mechanical information; and the unmyelinated nerve endings, or free nerve endings that register balance in the autonomic nervous system. Conscious touch and gentle traction or stretching induce relaxation and activate the parasympathetic nervous system. Because the whole body and all its systems are connected through the fascia, the touch also activates the central nervous system, which is involved in the modulation of muscle tone as well as movement. As a result, the central nervous system is aroused and responds by encouraging muscles and organs to find an easier, or more relaxed, position. The whole body relaxes in a profoundly deep way because the neurofascial system has been treated as a whole. And this may give us some clues as to how to address chronic pain from a new paradigm.

My experience of how to address chronic pain using this new paradigm comes from being a practitioner of Zero Balancing. Zero Balancers are trained to use skilled or conscious touch with a focus on the bones and the ligaments of the foundation and semi-foundation joints of the low back, spine, hips, feet, and neck. What I have found is that by treating these particular joints, the body can be brought into deep relaxation and balance in a relatively short period of time. I believe this is because these particular ligaments hold many of the interoceptive nerves (the unmyelinated sensory nerves) that communicate directly through the fascia into the autonomic nervous system. Using conscious touch to address the neurofascial system in this way gives the body-mind a sense of deep relaxation as well as access to its brilliant design.

Going back to Dr. Ingber's findings that manual therapy can actually remodel the fascial matrix, or tensegrity, of the cells, we see that mechanics-driven or direct physical stimulation could one day replace or enhance drug-based treatments for pain.[32] With conscious touch we can rebalance the neurofascial system and create more optimal environments for each part of the body down to the individual cells within us. Whatever the cause of chronic pain, the neurofascial system needs to be balanced as a whole in order to experience relief.

Interesting Note: These amazing qualities of fascia enable it to be our sixth sense. In fact, it takes in more information than all our senses combined. Since the sensory nerves in fascia are the "ears" listening to the mechanical, electrical, and magnetic forces undulating throughout your body, fascia gives us the ability to sense whether a person or situation is safe. When you walk into a room full of people you do not know, why is it that you are drawn to a certain person and not another? It may be your fascia that is picking up this information or the energy of a person. Why is it that you can sense whether a situation feels right? Fascia enables us to sense things outside of us and inside of us. Some believe fascia holds our belief systems and maybe even our consciousness.

Case Study: Cattie

Cattie came to me seeking relief from long-standing chronic neck and shoulder pain. Exercise and chiropractic work helped her, yet the stubborn achiness and pain kept

---

32 Ingber, Donald. 1998 Jan. The Architecture of Life. *Scientific American; 278:* 48–57. Retrieved from http://time.arts.ucla.edu/Talks/Barcelona/Arch_Life.htm

returning. Her marriage was not going well, sleep was a problem, her digestion was off, and she had severe allergies. In the first few sessions, I balanced her whole body with attention to her neck and shoulders with myofascial release, both direct and indirect (see "Bodywork in the fascia," Chapter 5). I also used my skills in balancing the foundation and semi-foundation joints of the skeleton. She would get relief for several days, but then the pain would return. I realized that even though Cattie's fascia could be released and her bones and joints could be balanced, something else needed attention.

I decided to look more closely at her autonomic nervous system by noticing her breathing patterns. Her inhalations and exhalations were quite shallow. I asked Cattie if she was willing to become more aware of her breath. I cannot stress enough the importance of soft, slow deep breathing as a way to address many issues of imbalance and tension in the body. (See more about the importance of proper breathing in Chapters 9 and 13.) The diaphragm resides deep in the neurofascial system, so Cattie and I worked together on aligning the diaphragm and connecting it to the pelvic floor using breath exercises (See Steps 6 and 7, The Wave Breath and the Core Hug Breath, in Part 4.) The pelvic floor and the diaphragm form the perfect fascial container for the organs deep in the body's inner core. Often the inner dimensions of the core need attention, and the only way to reach these inner dimensions is through breath.

Because Cattie held deep tension in her organs, her inner core was stuck. I introduced her to the body's support that comes from the inner core and to the Core Hug breath. Using breath to release the arousal of the sympathetic nervous system, Cattie's parasympathetic nervous system was reactivated so alignment and balance between the systems could return. The stuck stress pattern began to release, and her internal organs were able to relax.

With breath and subtle movements, she was able to move parts of her fascial web that had been gripping her internal organs. After a few sessions of incorporating breath work, the Fascial Release and Zero Balancing treatments began to hold. Her neck and shoulder pain was reduced. In addition, Cattie was also able to communicate with her husband more clearly, and her digestion improved. She began to actively treat her allergies through conventional and alternative methods. She developed a sparkle in her eyes and a lightness in her body. At home, she practiced lying on the roller and connecting to the breath and the deep inner core. Her neurofascial system was balancing. The more I work with the fascial and neurological systems together, the more I see how important they are in addressing chronic pain.

Chapter 8

Chronic Pain case studies

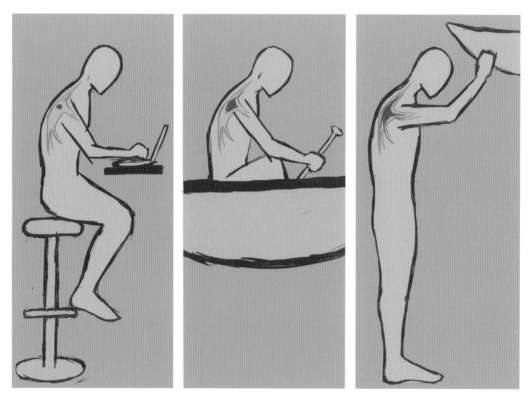

Acute chronic pain—The first two illustrations show a client hunched over a computer and hunched while rowing. Over the years, his fascial net took on this shape. When he went to lift a kayak in this misaligned state, his shoulder joint took the brunt and he experienced sudden pain.

Case Study: Jim—Chronic Pain That Comes on Suddenly

Many of my clients come to me for chronic pain that has come on suddenly (acute chronic pain). For example, Jim, forty-five years old, came to my office complaining of shoulder pain. He was a college dean who spent a good part of his day at the computer and on the phone. His weekends were spent doing a sport he loves, ocean rowing. He completed a 400-mile rowing race and had done well. After the race was over, Jim lifted his boat up onto the top of his car and suddenly felt a strong pain in his right shoulder. That one movement caused him to experience acute pain, but it was actually an accumulation of being in a forward posture at work and in his boat for many days, months, even years. Although the pain came on suddenly from this one event, it did not mean it was acute pain from this one event only. This is a type of chronic pain that has been building slowly in the body over time because the fascial net has been compromised. When Jim went to the doctor, he learned he had a rotator cuff injury. The doctor referred him to a physical therapist, but the treatments and exercises did not resolve his shoulder pain.

Upon taking Jim's history, I learned that had he had broken his right collarbone in a soccer game when he was thirteen years old. He had not received any treatment for the break, but through my visual and hands-on assessment of his shoulders, I felt the right shoulder had healed slightly forward. This slight misalignment created compensation patterns in Jim's facial web. It was barely noticeable when looking at him, but with my hands I could feel the forward placement in his fascial net that pulled his right shoulder in and down. The compensation pattern that began years ago was reinforced by his sitting in a forward slump at work and rowing in that posture on weekends.

During evaluation and assessment, I saw that Jim's whole right side was in a compromised pattern and that he was not using his fascial architecture as efficiently as he could. He was very strong, but he was out of alignment and disconnected from some of the support his architecture is designed to give him. By addressing the pattern throughout the architecture of the fascia and teaching him how to use his architectural support within him, his right shoulder realigned. Once in alignment, I taught Jim how to sustain his shoulder alignment himself by balancing on a soft foam roller. Once he could sustain his body alignment using his inner core architecture, he did shoulder strengthening exercises he learned from his physical therapist. The reason the strain in the rotator cuff muscles resolved was because he was now strengthening his shoulder in the proper alignment.

We worked together to help him be more aware of how he was sitting at work and in the boat. When the body is used well, is aligned, and the fascia is rehydrated, chronic pain melts out of the fascial net. So, when we consistently use our bodies efficiently, the fascia is fit and healthy enough to rebound back to a more optimal balance.

Case Study: Donna—Chronic Pain That Comes on Slowly

In most cases, I have clients who come to me for chronic pain that has come on slowly. Donna, fifty-five years old, a preschool teacher and administrator, arrived at my office after seeing several doctors, a physical therapist, and a chiropractor for back pain that had become increasingly worse over the years. Her doctor thought she needed surgery. What had started several years back as an occasional stiffness and soreness was now a throbbing sensation with occasional tingling down her left leg.

She was having trouble sleeping, and her moods were frequently irritable. Pain uses up a lot of energy. Bending down at work to help her small preschoolers was becoming more and more difficult. She had ignored her pain for years, managing it with anti-inflammatory medications when it got bad. She joined a gym to see if working out relieved the pain, but the relief was only temporary. She now knew her pain had become chronic and wanted to do something about it.

Upon taking Donna's history and assessing her structure, it was clear that a serious foot injury in a skiing accident in her early twenties was the original imprint of imbalance into her fascial net. She shared that her foot had healed well, but that it sometimes gave her trouble over the years. She thought nothing of it.

When I assessed her fascial architecture, it was noticeable that she had lost connection with her center of gravity in her fascial net, and her body was challenged in supporting itself in alignment. Using range-of-motion assessments of the foundation and semi-foundation joints and feeling for areas of hardened, stuck fascia, I surmised that Donna's back pain came from the misalignment of the foundation joints of her foot and the compensation patterns that had developed because of that misalignment. As a Zero Balancer, I learned that when foundation and semi-foundation joints are out of balance, the body cannot correct them on its own and compensates around the imbalance. Since these joints are below our conscious awareness, we do not realize how much compensating the body is doing. The whole spine, which needs deep fascial architecture for support, was out of balance and could not find its way back to that support. It had been straining and compensating for a long time and was at its breaking point. Could we possibly prevent the need for Donna to have surgery?

First, I worked with Donna to balance the foundation and semi-foundation joints of the spine and feet within the deeper fascial layers of ligaments and bone. These are where the dynamic ligaments that signal into the deep autonomic nervous system reside. Using myofascial release techniques, I released areas of stuck fascia in order to increase its suppleness and rehydrate the tissues. Then I shared with Donna the Sustainable Body training, which taught her how to connect to the center of gravity in the fascial web and then activate her inner core so she could sustain the work we did on the table. Without this training, the body often falls back into its compensation patterns. We made sure Donna kept the foundation joints of her foot where the original imprint occurred in balance by using a tennis ball exercise. (See Chapter 12 or Step 2 in Part 4.) She slowly built up the architectural support from within so she could sustain this alignment. It took a while, but she slowly regained the support and stability her low back needed to resolve her chronic pain.

Chronic Pain Resides in the Fascial Web

Jim is an example of chronic pain that comes on suddenly. Donna is an example of chronic pain that comes on slowly over time. Both cases indicate that in some way the fascial web has been misaligned and strained. The body is not able to rebalance itself, and compensation patterns develop as a response to the strains and pulls on the web. This shows up as chronic pain. The good news is that chronic pain can be treated if the body is viewed as a whole system. The bones can be balanced, and the fascial web can be remodeled back into a more optimal shape. The fluidity of the fascia can be treated so that it can communicate optimal alignment and balance throughout the system. The alignment and balance can be sustained using Sustainable Body training.

Freedom from Chronic Pain

We are one continuous fascial web, from birth to death, head to toe, skin to bone, organ to cell. We've learned that the connective tissue called fascia holds our body's shape, holds our physical and emotional imprints, communicates these imprints, and can be melted back into alignment. We've learned that tensegrity is a model for how our body holds itself up through a balance of tensions and can distribute strain throughout the body and enable us to be resilient in movement and in life. We've also learned that the fascia has its own communication system, the neurofascial system, which uses sensory nerves to register our alignment and misalignment, the homeostasis of our organs, and the spaces in our body.

The real-life examples of Steve, Cattie, Jim, and Donna show that most chronic pain results from imbalances in the neurofascial system. Our fascial net can be disturbed by surgery, jarred by injuries, imprinted by trauma, and weighed down by life. Whether chronic pain comes on suddenly or slowly, if we look more closely at the whole net and the connections within it, we may be able to find some answers—and some relief.

As Judy Foreman states in *A Nation in Pain,* we are in the "midst of a chronic pain epidemic," which is affecting over one hundred million American adults and costing the medical system billions of dollars.[33] As the baby boomer generation ages, it will cost even more. Pain that goes on for long periods of time creates such havoc in the nervous system that doing daily activities like sitting, standing, and walking are difficult and life is no longer fun. It has been documented that chronic pain can actually shrink the brain. Chronic pain is a whole new problem that affects us "biologically, psychologically, and socially."[34]

The good news is that there is hope. We just might be on the cusp of being able to treat chronic pain more effectively if we look at the body and the neurofascial system within it as a whole. Since the fascial fabric is primarily fluid and so ubiquitous, wrapping and weaving through everything, we now have a way to understand how all body movement can be transferred through the whole body in a seamless and unified way.

---

33 Foreman, Judy. (2014). *A Nation in Pain.* Oxford University Press, p. 1.
34 Foreman, Judy. (2014). *A Nation in Pain.* Oxford University Press, p. 4.

What would happen if we realign and rehydrate this fluid fascial fabric? What would happen if old injuries and compensation patterns are removed from the fascial web and then we reconnected to our natural balance and alignment? What would happen if we paid more attention to our fascia, its interconnections, its alignment and its fluidity? What if we embodied this new paradigm for understanding our bodies? What if we open to the possibility of living and moving within this system in harmony with the way it is designed without any shearing forces disturbing the health and resilience of our tissues? What if we could reclaim our "kid body," the natural way we used to move as children? Might more possibilities for well-being, health, vibrancy, and ease unfold? Our fascia is there to help us, so let's use it!

CHAPTER 9

THE CORE HUG:
HOW THE BODY ORGANIZES
AROUND A SINGLE POINT

The design of the human body, both structurally and energetically, is exquisite. The body's seamless nets, dynamic webs, folded layers with spaces in between bones and muscles, bridges, domes, and myofascial cables of connection reveal a design that is stable and versatile. The body's ability to respond to each nuanced movement we make and remain stable and balanced while we negotiate life's forces is a miracle. The more I learn about fascia, bone, and movement, the more I see the brilliant design within us. And the more I work with this design, the more I realize its role in relieving chronic pain for us all.

Embryology

Embryology, the study of the development of the embryo, may give us some insight on how our brilliant design starts to form.[35] In the first weeks of life, cells divide repeatedly from a single point of origin. The cells organize around a point. At about two weeks into the embryo's development, the connective tissue cells (fascial stem cells, if you will) start giving signals that help cells differentiate their individual jobs. Every body part needs a container in which to form. The fascial cells create the containers and spaces for some cells to develop into the brain, others into the bones, the muscles, and the different organs. This is the earliest fluid state of what becomes our connective tissue or fascial

---

35 Myers, Thomas. 2014. *Anatomy Trains: Myofascial Meridians for Manual and Movement Therapists, 3rd Edition,* Churchill Livingstone, pp. 36–38.

body. As development continues, the embryo folds and grows within layers of the continuum. There is a folding and refolding of layers in the body, a process called "double bagging," which becomes the body's seamless fascial web. The spaces between the bags form the three different nets—the neural, circulatory, and fascial nets—that give our bodies their shape. Powerful spirals and vortexes of movement give rise to complex form. As the embryo continues to grow, it keeps folding like a body-wide origami until the last folds occur in the roof of the mouth. Cleft palate is a condition where the last folds of the origami go awry. As this double bagging is occurring, the body is organizing around a line. Using this embryological theory of how the body organizes itself—around a single point and around a single line—we can delve into how to work with and embody this body-wide net of support.

The Myth of the Core

If you have ever taken a fitness class or worked with a trainer, you have probably been told to do core exercises. It is now very popular to teach exercises that revolve around strengthening the core. However, these programs tend to use the term "core" to mean the abdominal muscles. Strong abs or developing a "six pack" is the goal. Our obsession with having strong abdominal muscles actually binds up the diaphragm and creates a fight-or-flight stress response that keeps us in a low-grade chronic tense state. We are not aware of this because this chronic tension has become our norm. Unfortunately, we no longer know what it feels like to be fully relaxed. Our belly is tightly held. We do not know how to feel a deeper sense of the core as an all-body phenomenon.

I will try to keep things simple here. Fitness books line the shelves with programs to strengthen your core doing sit-ups and planks. Excellent books have been written about the design of the bones and muscles and fascia in the bodywork and movement field, and I encourage you to seek out the wealth of information available.

However, what I want to emphasize here is that because of embryology—the body's folding and refolding of itself—and the liquid brilliance of the connective tissue, the core is much more complex than we think. To simplify this complexity, let's think of the core myofascia as forming two layers: an inner layer, or inner corset, that has direct connections to the spine and organs, and a more superficial layer, or outer corset, that does not. Healthy alignment depends on you being able to distinguish between the two layers of core support.[36] Most fitness and rehabilitation programs overemphasize the outer layer of the core muscles, which is easy to feel, so that makes strengthening them easy to teach. Unfortunately, outer core work can easily overwhelm the inner core, thus making it weaker. If we only strengthen our abdominal muscles, the myofascia designed to support the spine can become weaker. It is possible to do too much core work. When we overwork, our muscles get tight and the core cannot breathe. If the core is forced into the inner layers, we lose the freedom of movement that is necessary for graceful posture, ease of movement, and refined awareness of structural support from the inner core.

Less Is More

To connect to the inner core layer, it is important to *feel* the connections within the bones, muscles, and fascia of the body in a more subtle way. It is important to relax and breathe to connect to the core. To do less and feel more is counterintuitive to most of our concepts of fitness, but "less is more" is important in this case. If we think of the fascia as an organ of innerness, this makes sense.

The body is designed with two kinds of muscle fibers: fast-twitch fibers and slow-twitch fibers. Fast-twitch fibers contract quickly and tire rapidly. We use these fibers when our muscles need to be used for strength or a sudden activity. These are the fibers in the outer core muscles. Slow-twitch fibers are designed to sustain continuous muscle tension, and they do this without tiring. These fibers are designed to hold a perfect balance of muscle tension—remember tensegrity—for our stability. I like to imagine these fibers as the ones that hug the body from the inside out. Even though the inner core is composed of both fast- and slow-twitch fibers, a greater number of slow-twitch fibers live in the inner core layer.

---

36 Bond, Mary. 2006. *The New Rules of Posture: How to Sit, Stand, and Move in the Modern World.* Healing Arts Press.

Optimal posture depends on the connections of these slow-twitch fibers within the myofascia of the inner core. In Part 4 you will learn how to connect to the inner core through breath and how to connect the slow-twitch fibers of the deep myofascial core using subtle movement. If you connect to the center of gravity deep in the belly and then bring in the inner core slow-twitch fibers of the Vertical Core into connection, you are reconnecting into the neurofascial system. This is an avenue for relieving chronic pain.

The Center of Gravity

I am inspired by the illustration of the Vitruvian Man by Leonardo da Vinci. The image, which da Vinci drew around 1490, provides an understanding of human proportions and represents his attempts to relate man to nature. Taking the concepts of the architect, Vitruvius, he found the exact center of the human body. We call it the center of gravity. I call it the Core Hug. I believe it is the center of the fascial web.

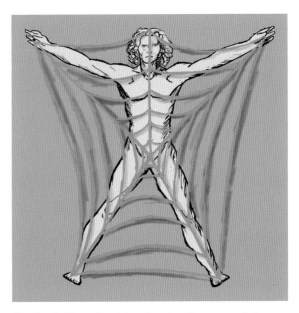

da Vinci's Vitruvian Man showing the center of the fascial web

The center of gravity in the body is defined as the balancing point where the body can be in equilibrium, or a point where the sum of all the forces and movements acting on the body is zero. It is the point at which the weight of the body rests and from which all the parts balance. Using Western anatomy and Eastern energy theory, it is located in the front of the sacrum at the second sacral vertebra. As we moved from being horizontal, four-legged beings to vertical, upright beings, the stimulation on the bones at the base of the spine resulted in our sacral bones fusing together as a response to the weight of our body in the upright position.

Due to the forces of gravity on the bones and the fascia around them, our bodies built up bone to strengthen and stabilize the pelvis and the pelvic floor of fascia to suspend those bones for our vertical structures. This is a theoretical center, because the center is not stationary. It is continually shifting as we walk and move in space. Our fascia allows our center of gravity to shift in an infinite number of ways and still keeps us dynamically stable. Yet when we are standing upright, our center of gravity tends to remain at or near the sacrum.

The first person to show us the center of gravity in the human body was not da Vinci. Hundreds of years earlier, civilizations emphasized this center of gravity in the human body. Chinese medicine calls this center "*dantian*," meaning "the root of the tree of life." It is considered to be the foundation of rooted standing, breathing, and body awareness in qigong and all martial arts. The term is often interchangeable with the Japanese word "*hara*," which

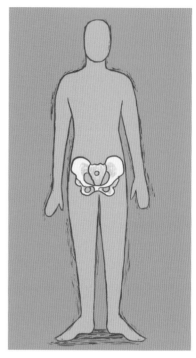

The center of gravity in the upright body is located two inches in front of the base of the spine.

means belly. In Chinese, Korean, and Japanese traditions it is considered the physical center of gravity of the human body and the seat of one's internal energy. In yoga philosophy, it is thought to be the seat of *prana*, which radiates outwards to the entire body. Most movement teachers, dancers, and professional athletes must know this center well. Sue Hitzmann, the person behind the MELT Method, calls it the body's GPS.[37] I call it the Core Hug. This is the point around which the body organizes and navigates the forces that move through us. Without this signal from the body's center, the body has a challenging time organizing itself for alignment and balance. When we connect to this point, the fascial web organizes itself more efficiently.

---

37 Hitzmann, Sue. 2013. *The MELT Method: A Breakthrough Self-Treatment System to Eliminate Chronic Pain, Erase the Signs of Aging, and Feel Fantastic in Just 10 Minutes a Day!* New York, Harper Collins.

The Importance of Breath

Maybe you realize that you do not breathe correctly, but you don't know how to change your breathing habits. Join the club! In our society, it seems like physical fitness and exercise keep us on the fast track and keep us in dysfunctional breathing patterns. As you strain through your core workout, push through a yoga pose or Pilates move, you may be reminded to breathe. But are you breathing with the correct muscles? If not, you have lost connection to your true center. Unfortunately, the center of gravity gets lost in the training of the outer core and the movement muscles as we do sit-ups, planks, leg raises, and Russian twists. This is because connecting to the center of gravity involves being still and breathing fully from the deep soft belly. You are not strengthening your breathing patterns by cardio workouts. Your heart may be getting a great workout, but your breathing muscles are not getting much of a workout at all. "All chronic pain, suffering, and disease is caused by a lack of oxygen at the cell level. . . . Proper breathing nourishes the cells of the body with oxygen, and optimizes the functioning of the body on all levels."[38] Stuck fascia prevents oxygen from getting to the cells. If there is one thing you can do for chronic pain, your alignment, and your health, learn to breathe in a way that is anatomically correct and harmonious with all your systems.

One of the most efficient ways to change your breathing patterns and find the center of gravity within the body is through breath, but not just any kind of breath. When you were a baby, you began your breath deep in your soft belly. Watch a baby breathe and notice how the belly moves up and down slowly and effortlessly. Due to life stresses, you lost your ability to soften the belly and begin the breath from deep in the center of the body. Somewhere along the line, your breathing went out of whack, but you are not aware of it or do not have ways to regain deep breathing patterns. In our fast-paced society, we live in the fight-or-flight shallow breathing pattern. No wonder there's an increase in chronic pain and sleep and digestive disorders.

Breathing the way your body was designed to do—centered in the middle of your body at your center of gravity—needs some retraining and attention to the anatomy of

---

38 Dr. Arthur C. Guyton, as cited in Vranich, Belisa. (2014). *Breathe: 14 days to oxygenating, recharging, and fueling your body & brain.* New York, Breathing Class Press, p. 7.

breathing. To relearn how to breathe, we need to go back to how we breathed as infants, which means moving the breath down to the lower part of your body, or belly breathing. The best breathing starts in the belly. The lower section of the ribs move, your belly expands, your side ribs widen, even your back expands. When you learn to regain the rest-and-digest breathing pattern, which is slower and deeper, you nourish and replenish the fascia in and around the organs, address the stuck fascia affecting your nervous system, and relieve chronic pain from deep within.

Dismantling breathing habits and replacing them with new habits takes practice and curiosity. As you practice belly breathing, don't think you have to breathe this way all the time. This is a just a way to bring in new breathing habits and recondition your breathing muscles and the neurofascial systems. Eventually, belly breathing will happen more naturally and more often.

The center of gravity is found in stillness. In this stillness and making a conscious commitment to fully exhale, the bones and the myofascia of the pelvis come together around the body's center of gravity. In this process, the belly can be trained to be toned and relaxed. The natural contraction that comes at the end of a full exhale activates the sensory nerve endings in the fascia that subtly hug your spine, pelvic floor, and organs from all sides. The deep core is hugged. This teaches you where the center of gravity in your body resides and how to use it to keep you aligned and pain-free.

As I teach people the Core Hug, I often hear statements like the ones below.

"I've been studying yoga for over twelve years, but Karen was the first person to ever truly show me the sensation of the bandhas [the activation of the deep core via the breath]." —Krista

"I remember my dance teacher always telling us to feel the core, but until I did the Core Hug breath, I never knew what she was talking about." —Danielle

Try It! The Core Hug Breath

There are several avenues you can use to practice the Core Hug breath. One way is to lie comfortably on the floor with your knees bent. Another way that enables you to feel the Core Hug breath more accurately and more three-dimensionally is to practice with a towel or yoga mat rolled the long way, a bolster, or a thirty-six-inch soft foam roller. You can use a firm foam roller, but place a thick towel, blanket, or yoga mat over it to create some softness and give. (See Chapter 1 to learn more about the roller.)

Step 1: Lie down comfortably on your back with your knees bent. To align the neck, place a folded towel or small pillow under your head.

You may use a prop (rolled up towel, yoga mat, or soft roller), but only if it is comfortable and supportive. Place the prop on the floor behind you vertically, sit on the end of the prop, and then roll your spine down onto it, from tailbone to the back of your head, keeping your knees bent. (See Part 4, Steps 4 and 11 for instructions on how to get on and off the roller safely.) To align your neck, place a folded towel or small pillow under your head.

Step 2: First, take a few soft, slow, deep breaths in and out through your nose. Now do the Wave Breath by imagining you are at the ocean watching the waves. Watch your breath begin deep in the ocean of your belly and flow gently up to the shore of your chest. Waves do not force themselves out of the ocean, nor do they push themselves onto the shore. Match each breath to the rhythm of a wave as you watch it arise out of your belly and flow onto the upper chest. (For step-by-step instructions to the Wave Breath, see Part 4, Step 6.) As you inhale, the diaphragm goes down to meet the pelvic floor. As you exhale, the diaphragm floats up, toward the roof of your mouth. All your organs are getting a massage. Find a soft, slow, even rhythm and notice that the body is finding its spaces as the movement of the breath nourishes the fascial tissues around the organs and deep in the center of the body. This breath prepares you for the Core Hug Breath.

Step 3: The Core Hug breath:
a) Take a soft, slow, deep inhalation through the nose, watching the breath begin in the deep, soft belly.
b) On the exhale, open your mouth, softly and slowly whisper to yourself, "La, la, la, la." Focus on getting all the air out until you can no longer utter a "la." This is committing to the end of the exhale. If you exhale fully, you will sense a slight activation as the navel moves toward the spine. I emphasize *slight* because it is not a tightening or

gripping of the abdominal muscles that you may be used to feeling. It is a subtle neurofascial engagement.

c) If you cannot feel the slight activation of your navel moving toward your spine, do the following: as you come to the end of the exhale and cannot utter one more "la," stick your tongue out and blow the remaining air out of your lungs. This should help you activate the center of gravity at the base of your spine.

d) Repeat until you feel the subtle contraction at the end of each exhale. If you feel your muscles tensing or gripping, release them. Let the breath do the work, not the muscles. Repeat four to five times. This is your first access point into the Core Hug.

Step 4: Adding dimensions to the Core Hug

a) With a soft, slow, deep breath and a commitment to the exhale, the body naturally pulls the pelvic bones toward each other. As you reach the end of the exhale, feel the subtle activation of the belly moving in towards the spine.

b) Now, very gently lift the pelvic floor (not a forceful Kegel squeeze, but a subtle lift). Simultaneously, gently press the sacrum (low back) into the floor or the roller, stabilizing your sacroiliac joints at the base of the spine.

c) These three dimensions of activation—bringing the bones and fascia of the pelvis together, up, and back—create a Core Hug at the center of the body.

d) It is important to keep your muscles relaxed; this is *not* a squeezing or tightening of muscles. Instead, feel a sensation of activation as the core hug connects you deeply to the center of your fascial web in the exact center of your body. With this signal activated, you give yourself a deep internal hug that sends signals out into the fascial web, from the deepest layer of bone out, to create the support that nourishes and restores your alignment and your health.

For step-by-step instructions to connect to your Core Hug breath, see Part 4, Step 7.

Case Study: Krista

Krista is an active woman who teaches yoga at a popular Boston yoga studio. She is experiencing pain in her back and hips, which is getting worse as her teaching schedule increases.

She finds herself pushing through yoga poses as she demonstrates them to her students. Krista had back surgery when she was in her early twenties and now wonders if the surgery may have created more problems. After surgery, scar tissue develops. Scar tissue is the fascia doing what it is meant to do: heal a tear or rip in the fascial fabric. Yet once the fabric is knitted back together, thick scar tissue can block the communication the fascia needs to negotiate stability and movement. When I evaluated her structure, we found that her outer core was quite strong, but her inner core was weak.

As Krista lay on the soft foam roller with her front body open and relaxed, I led her in simple breathing awareness, which helped her visualize and realign her diaphragm, and then connected her to her center of gravity and the pelvic floor. She became aware that she had no connection to her center of gravity, the Core Hug, even though she had a daily yoga practice.

MY SUSTAINABLE BODY STORY: KRISTA

"I had been experiencing chronic pain radiating from my low back to hips for years; [I] had seen chiropractors, orthopedics, and physical therapists with fragmented success. I am a yoga instructor, and the pain, caused especially when transitioning through vinyasa, was debilitating to my practice and livelihood, but also affected daily activities. I've been studying yoga for over twelve years, but Karen was the first person to ever truly show me the sensation of the bandhas (activation of the deep core via the breath). In our first session, she used a foam roller to connect me to the deep core, and then for the next hour and thirty minutes held space for me, as I released eight years of emotional and physical pain. I can't exactly explain how she heals, but the most important piece is that she guides you with a combination of techniques and innate intuition toward an intrinsic alignment of body, mind, and spirit."

What we learned is that Krista's surgery had created scar tissue that was blocking the neurofascial signals from the center of gravity. Her body needed these signals to orient from the center point and navigate the forces of gravity in the vertical body. I have found with myself and my clients that by balancing the body on the soft roller vertically, it is easier to feel the dimensions of the inner core and the center of gravity. Krista immediately noticed the difference between her inner and outer core muscles and was excited to feel that connection. She understood why she was having back and hip pain and was empowered with ways to reconnect to the center of gravity and the inner core. She now had hope that she could connect to that center point and find a new strength within. Krista had the tools to connect to and embody the Core Hug using her breath. From there, we were able to release the blockages in the scar tissue and reconnect Krista from the inner core out.

The Core Difference

The more I work with myself and my clients, the more I realize how few people truly sense the difference between the outer and inner core and where the center of gravity resides in the body. I have yoga, Pilates, dance, and fitness instructors comment with surprise that they have not been connected to the true center of gravity. They know the outer core well, but are not as acquainted with the inner core. All sorts of breathing patterns develop that keep us from connecting to the center of gravity. Instead of a toned but soft belly, we hold the belly tightly. Without this center, the Core Hug, our bodies flail about trying to negotiate gravity, but we are not doing it efficiently.

When we connect to our center of gravity, we have reconnected to the single point around which our body organizes itself. We are going back to the original movement that occurred as we formed from an embryo into the beautifully designed beings that we are.

CHAPTER 10

THE VERTICAL CORE: HOW THE BODY ORGANIZES AROUND A LINE

Since we are vertical structures, in addition to this center of gravity in the pelvis the body also organizes around a vertical axis or line. My hypothesis is that the vertical line in the body consists of four guidewires of myofascia (vertical lines of fascia and muscles) that I call the Vertical Core, or inner core. Two guidewires, the Deep Front Line, run up the front of the body from the inner arches of the feet to the jaw; the other two guidewires, the Deep Back Line, run up the back of the body from the arches of the feet to the back of the head. Because these guidewires connect to the foundation and semi-foundation joints in the feet, low back, and spine, they are key to supporting and suspending the bones, and thus the entire body.

Remember embryology: after two weeks of embryonic development, the cells start to organize around a line as the layers of fascial tissue fold and refold within the body as it double bags itself. The vertical body uses this framework with its different layers to communicate and transmit forces. The skeleton and the fascial wrapping around the bones is the deepest and densest layer in the folding. According to the Working Energy Model used by Dr. Fritz Smith, this is the layer through which the strongest currents are transmitted from our feet grounded on the earth to our skull, which connects us to the sky.

The next layer of soft tissues closest to the bones, the body's soft tissue skeleton, consists of myofascia: ligaments, tendons, muscles, and internal organs. Together the bones of the skeleton and deeper soft tissue skeleton transmit the forces from the deepest layer out as we sit, stand, walk, and move in the world. When we move using our center of gravity and vertical axis of myofascia, we transfer weight from side to side, front to back, and oblique to oblique evenly and elastically. Oblique force fields and figure eight patterns are created when we walk. A balanced body is orienting around an ever-changing center of gravity within the pelvic bowl.[39] Since we are vertical beings, we need to transmit the forces of gravity through our vertical structures efficiently.

The Body's Guidewires of Support

Imagine your spine is your body's deep vertical telephone pole or sail mast. Neither the telephone pole nor the sail mast can hold itself up in gravity. The support for the spine is found in the deeper layers of myofascia that form a column of support for the spine, or the midline of the body. These are the body's guidewires—the body's soft tissue skeleton. I am proposing that the guidewires for our vertical, two-legged structure are the myofascial meridians of Tom Myers's Deep Front Line and Yaron Gal Carmel's Deep Back Line. These myofascial meridians support the Vertical Core, (the inner core) of the human structure. These fascial guidewires—two in the front of the body and two in the back of the body—need to be balanced and connected to the body's center of gravity and communicating efficiently through the myofascia of the inner core in order to hold the body up and stabilize it for movement. These guidewires are not static, but dynamically fluid to negotiate our movements. A guidewire, or guy-wire, is defined as "a tensioned cable designed to add stability to a freestanding structure. They are used commonly in ship masts, radio masts, wind turbines, utility poles, fire service extension ladders, and are also used in church raises and tents."[40] Your body's guidewires, when balanced and aligned, are perfectly tensioned cables that hold you up effortlessly.

Guidewires for the front body

Let's look at the Deep Front Line first. This myofascial meridian is the deepest and takes up more volume in the body than any of the other lines Myers has mapped. It runs up the front on both sides of the body and forms the body's myofascial Vertical Core. This

---

39 Smith, Fritz Frederick, MD. 1986. *Inner Bridges: A Guide to Energy Movement and Body Structure. Atlanta, GA: Humanics Limited.* p. 29.
40 https://en.wikipedia.org/wiki/Guy-wire

line begins deep in the underside of the foot, up the inseam of the lower leg, and behind the knee to inside of the thigh. From here, the line passes in front of the hip joint, pelvis, and spine up through the diaphragm and rib cage, through the thoracic viscera and front of the neck, ending on the underside of the jaw and the side of the head. These two dynamic guidewires of the Deep Front Line take up a lot of space in the body.

The Deep Front Line contains many of the unconscious, slow-twitch fibers of the inner core that are designed for stability. According to Myers,[41] this line is key to posture and alignment because it:

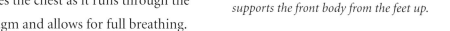

The vertical Deep Front Line of myofascia that supports the front body from the feet up.

1. Supports the feet as it lifts the inner arches.
2. Stabilizes each segment of the legs: ankles, knees, groin.
3. Supports the lumbar spine from the front and affects the rhythm of walking.
4. Stabilizes the chest as it runs through the diaphragm and allows for full breathing.
5. Balances the neck and head on top of the spine.
6. Links with the sympathetic, parasympathetic, and enteric nervous systems and responds to stress and relaxation because of its proximity to the organs.

The trauma line

Since the Deep Front Line lies deep within the body and connects with key joints in the skeleton, it links the structural and energetic core of the body. This line also

---

41 Myers, Thomas. 2014. *Anatomy Trains: Myofascial Meridians for Manual and Movement Therapists, 3rd Edition,* Churchill Livingstone.

connects to our center of gravity and forms a large part of the inner core. Because of its location near major organs, it affects the circulatory, respiratory, digestive, and reproductive systems. The key to homeostasis within the body is balance between the sympathetic (stress) nervous system and the parasympathetic (rest) nervous system (see Chapter 7). When we experience stress or trauma, this line will be affected. Because of its intimate connection to the neurofascial system, it communicates and holds the body's reactions to stress and trauma: fight, flight, or freeze. Some call this the trauma line. This grand line roots our feet, creates our internal core support, lifts us out of the forces of gravity, and supports our vertical balance and the body's suspension system.

As Earls and Myers emphasize in their book *Fascial Release for Structure Balance*, "the importance of the Deep Front Line to posture, movement, and attitude cannot be overemphasized. A dimensional understanding of this line is necessary for successful application of nearly any method of manual or movement therapy. . . . Restoration of the

MY SUSTAINABLE BODY STORY: RELEASING TRAUMA IN THE DEEP FRONT LINE

During my Structural Strategies training with Tom Myers, I had the opportunity to be a model for the class. As a model, I give permission to be analyzed in front of the class for structural imbalances. This gives my fellow students a chance to practice developing strategies for treatment. When Tom looked at my structure, he noticed two things. The first was my feet; I have high arches. He respectfully commented, "At some point in Karen's life, most likely it was a time before she could talk, 'preverbal,' her feet took on the message: I want to get out of here!"

As a child growing up in an unsafe household, there must have been many times I wanted to get out of a tense situation, but I could not. Tom's observation rang true somewhere inside of me. The second thing Tom noticed was that my Deep Front Line was twisted to the right like a corkscrew, starting at the feet to the middle of the heart/lung/chest area. Now that I am better versed in the Deep Front Line, I see that my issues are related to this line, which begins in the feet and runs up through my deep inner core, the places where my trauma is held.

After completing the Structural Strategies training with Tom, and incorporating it into my treatment protocol, my practice thrived. I was balancing parenting, dissolving my marriage, and working with more and more clients. The fascial armor I had built up to protect me in an unsafe marriage was thawing, my yoga practice was not as solid, so my shoulder pain was becoming chronic. My body hurt. I had been "Rolfed" by my previous teacher in years past. It was time to commit to another ten-session series of Rolfing. I began the series with Yaron Gal Carmel, one of the first practitioners trained in Tom Myers' Anatomy Trains Myofascial Meridian series. Yaron brings a mechanical engineering background to his in-depth understanding of anatomy and physiology. Yaron is a grounded, heart-centered practitioner with integrity. I was glad to be in his hands for the series.

CONNECTED HEAD TO TOE

Yaron followed the ten-session series protocol, beginning with the superficial lines in the early sessions and the Deep Front Line, which is divided into two sessions in the middle of the series. Most of the time I was able to take in the work, but I remember how painful it was when he worked on my feet.

Session seven, which treats the neck and mouth, stands out for me. This session is designed to work on the end of the Deep Front Line. It is important to mention here that during this process, I had developed a trust for Yaron as a practitioner. This is crucial for any type of release to happen with any style of bodywork one is receiving. In this session, I began to feel a clear connection between the inner arches of my feet and my neck and mouth. It was clear how the fascia in my neck and mouth at the end of the Deep Front Line was directly connected to my inner arches.

Then I felt connections deep into the center of my chest/lung area. My breathing altered. The deep myofascial core cylinder that Tom had observed twisted like a corkscrew began to unwind.

Waves of energy pulsated through as my neck and mouth were worked by Yaron's sensitive hands and conscious touch. A deep feeling of grief rose into my consciousness. As the grief surfaced, I did not avoid it or run away from it. I was supported and grounded from below, in my feet. My Deep Front Line was connecting from my arches to my head. I could feel the deep inner core support. I felt safe! I began to repeat to myself, "I am safe. I am safe. I am safe." Then I said it out loud over and over again. Yaron stayed present and his hands and words held me. The need to twist myself up like a corkscrew as my strategy not to feel fear, anxiety, lack of safety, anger, and hurt began to unwind itself. My inner trauma core was realigning and resetting itself. As deep grief surfaced, waves of gratitude poured through me. I felt the presence of support in my life—friends, family, colleagues, healing practitioners, my teachers, God. It was profoundly healing.

proper DFL functioning is by far the best preventative measure for structural and movement therapies."[42]

Read more about trauma and the neurofascial system's response in Chapter 11.

Guidewires for the back body

Now let's look at the Deep Back Line. This line was mapped more recently by Yaron, who is now a senior faculty member at Kinesis School of Structural Integration and an expert in anatomy and physiology in his own right. Yaron pursued his investigation of

---

42 Earls, James, and Myers, Thomas. (2010). *Fascial Release for Structural Balance*. Lotus Publishing and North Atlantic Books. p. 274)

Tom's myofascial meridians asking whether there might be a counterforce to the Deep Front Line. He explored this question using the principles of tensegrity, biotensegrity, embryology, and his work with clients. When he participated in a week-long dissection workshop at Tufts Medical School with one of the leaders in the field of fascial medicine, his hypothesis was reinforced and his discovery of the Deep Back Line came to the fore. When Yaron introduced me to the Deep Back Line, as a Zero Balancing practitioner, I was struck by its direct correlation to the foundation and semi-foundation joints of the skeleton. As a result, this line of myofascia has become a crucial component of my work.[43]

The Deep Back Line also begins in the inner arch of the foot and runs parallel to the Deep Front Line up the inseam of the leg, up through the pelvis in the back body, low back, and upper back to the neck, ending in the forehead. It also connects to the center of gravity and the pelvic floor. It embraces the deep fascia of the spine and the brain. Deep fascial elements of the Deep Front Line affect the organs and the breath, the Deep Back Line also affects the deep fascia of all the bones and joints along the spine, which also connect to the sympathetic and parasympathetic nervous systems. Yaron has posited that the intricate connections along this line ending at the back of the neck could also be registering our reaction to trauma and stress—our startle reflex. Through the course of evolution, the startle reflex has played an important part in producing forces in these tissues that communicate to the brain and the pituitary to protect us from attack or stress (see Chapter 11).

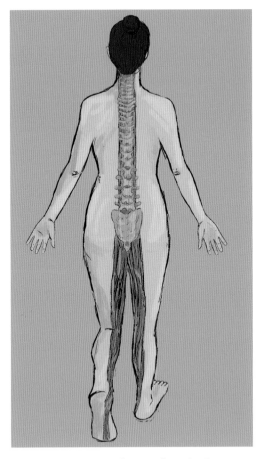

The vertical Deep Back Line of myofascia supports the back body from the feet up.

---

43 Carmel, Yaron Gal. 2014. *The Deep Back Line and a Proposed Alternate Superficial Back Line.* International Association of Structural Integrators Yearbook.

The Vertical Core

By understanding the guidewires of the Deep Front Line and Deep Back Line, we now have a vertical line around which the body organizes itself for movement. I imagine the four guidewires coming together to form a fascial column of support designed to hold up the vertical skeleton in a balance of tension between bones and fascia. This dynamic column is the Vertical Core. Together these four guidewires form a column of support and transmit the vertical forces that move through us. When these vertical guidewires are balanced and connected, the strongest energy currents can flow through our bones, and the liquid brilliance of the fascia can support every movement we make. We are supported and aligned effortlessly.

As the fiber optics of our body's deep internet, when these fibrous cables get frayed or cut, sheared or stressed, the whole body goes into compensation for the loss of support these guidewires provide. When the skeleton loses its vertical balance, so do these guidewires. We lose connection to the design of our bones and our fascial guidewires that hold us up. We lose our biotensegrity from within. Our spine's telephone pole or sail mast gets pulled down with the forces of gravity. We are not able to work with gravity because we have lost the design that buoys us up out of gravity. Our parts do not work together, our joints get stuck, the ligaments and tendons shear, the muscles overwork, and the fascial web loses its ability to communicate through the fiber optics of the guidewires. This is the perfect storm for chronic pain to manifest. If we balance the bones, get these myofascial guidewires back online, and get these parts communicating with each other, then we can realign the body and move out of chronic pain and into ease and grace.

The iliopsoas: the most important part of your vertical core from the front

The Vertical Core supports the front body using the Deep Front Line. Located in the midsection of this Line is the most important skeletal muscle in the human body: the iliopsoas muscle. Located near the center of gravity, the iliopsoas is the only muscle that connects the upper and lower body. All other muscles are either lower or upper body muscles. Not this one! It is the body's center of power, movement, and balance. Its location affects posture, balance, walking, energy, nerves, and emotions. The importance of this muscle and its connection to how the body functions cannot be overemphasized.

The iliopsoas consists of two muscles: the psoas (major and minor) and the iliacus. The psoas major is deep within the front of the hip joint and attaches to the lower spine. The psoas minor connects the pelvis to the spine and is less important since we walk on two legs instead of four. The iliacus runs from the inner thigh to the iliac bone of the pelvis. This group of muscles flexes the hip, is the deepest of the hip flexors, and possibly the strongest as a muscle group. Sources state that because of the location, the iliacus acts on the pelvis and the psoas acts on the spine. For my purposes here, I would like to single out the psoas because of its job in stabilizing the low back. The psoas is made of many slow-twitch fibers that hug the lower spine for support. As we walk, or when we reach up to get something from a high shelf, the psoas stabilizes the low back. When people talk about your hip flexors, I wonder if they realize that not only does this important muscle act as a prime mover, but it's a critical stabilizer of the spine as well. We have overlooked its importance in stabilization and its ability to affect posture.

When I talk about fascia and the inner core, please realize that no one muscle works alone. The inner core is a group of muscles and fascia, or myofascia, that girdle the spine and hold it in balance. When all the muscles of the inner core are working together and connected, the body senses its alignment. We connect to another layer of our strength, which is often a layer we are less familiar with. This connection to our deeper strength allows the outer core and muscular effort to release and relax.

The psoas is not an abdominal muscle. It is an inner core muscle. It acts as "a keystone, central and superior to the 'flying buttresses' of the femurs and thigh muscles. This major architectural concept is also apparent in the skeletal pelvis/leg relationship, and supports the human body much like an arch does in building structures," explains JoAnn Staugaard-Jones in her book, *The Vital Psoas Muscle: Connecting Physical,*

Emotional, and Spiritual Well-Being.[44] As a skeletal muscle that works two joints, the psoas has another role: it acts as a shelf, "supporting internal organs, along with the pelvis as a basin, and the pelvic floor."[45] Traveling vertically along the guidewires, the psoas connects the spine to the leg. Traveling through the center of gravity, it connects the guidewires to each other. It transmits forces and is responsible for fluid movement. It is responsible for so much that making sure it functions correctly is important to your health. If it is too tight and stressed from doing a lot of repetitive movement, it becomes exhausted and imbalanced. It needs to be relaxed, supple, hydrated, and connected.

The "muscle of trust"

Because of the fascial connections and location near the organs, the psoas affects the circulatory system (heart), the digestive system (intestines, excretion/elimination), detoxification (liver, kidneys), respiratory system (diaphragm), and the reproductive system (male and female reproductive organs). It also affects energy flow through the body and holds deep emotional imprints due to our responses to gut feelings, stress, and safety. I learned early in my bodywork career to call the iliopsoas "the muscle of trust." This is why the Deep Front Line is also called the "trauma line." If we experience fear or trauma, we either fight, run, or curl up into a ball. This is the muscle that allows us to do those movements. This muscle is intimately connected to the neurofascial system signaling homeostasis or imbalance in the autonomic nervous system. It is also part of our fascia's interoception system that perceives balance or imbalance within the organs of our deep inner core. This is why connecting and freeing the psoas gently and mindfully with breath and gentle stretching is crucial to full body health. (For exercises to connect to the breath and lengthen the psoas, see Part 4, Step 13, Opening Hip Fans.)

---

44 Staugaard-Jones, JoAnn. (2012.) *The Vital Psoas Muscle: Connecting Physical, Emotional, and Spiritual Well-Being. Berkeley, CA: North Atlantic Books.*
45 Staugaard-Jones, JoAnn. (2012.) *The Vital Psoas Muscle: Connecting Physical, Emotional, and Spiritual Well-Being. Berkeley, CA: North Atlantic Books.*

I encourage you to find a good hands-on practitioner, movement educator, or yoga or Pilates teacher who has knowledge and expertise in treating the psoas. With trustworthy support, you can accelerate your connections and healing of this deep inner core muscle. The main thing is to be gentle, do not push, relax, breathe, go slowly, and move with tenderness toward your inner core.

MY SUSTAINABLE BODY STORY: DEBORAH R.

I developed various irregular heartbeat patterns that began to emerge in my sixties and became more problematic as time passed. After my physical therapist realized that my left lung did not exhale properly and my left rib cage was not open, Karen started honing in on that problem. She eventually identified a mass of scar tissue/fascia that was likely interfering with my vagus nerve and touching off the heart arrhythmias. So, for the past year, Karen and I have been focusing on my chest, rib cage, the scar tissue, and muscle groups related to firing up the Vertical Core guidewires that Karen's work identifies and strengthens. Given that my issues likely stemmed from injuries related to preverbal trauma, my healing has touched all levels of my emotional, physical, and energetic/spiritual body.

The low back: the most important part of your vertical core from the back

The Vertical Core supports the back body using the Deep Back Line. Key muscles and joints in the midsection of this line support you from the back. The psoas is also connected with the low back because it attaches to the sides of the five lumbar vertebrae. Along with the psoas, the low back and pelvic area is an elaborate architecture of bones, ligaments, muscles, and nerves designed to support you from the center of gravity out to all other parts of the body. To function properly, these areas must be in balance and alignment with each other. If this major area of the body is out of balance or misaligned, it will affect the rest of the spine, the hips, the feet, the neck, and even the jaw. Essentially, the entire length of the Vertical Core in the body is affected, and the low back especially.

Low back pain has become a "disease" in its own right. According to Foreman's analysis, chronic low back pain is the fifth most common reason for doctor visits, costs millions in lost work days, and billions of dollars have been spent on new interventions and thousands of studies.[46] Interventions such as electrical stimulation, transcranial magnetic stimulation, nerve blocks, steroids, Botox, nerve killing, and surgery for low back pain may not relieve the pain. Evidence suggests that noninvasive treatments should be tried before considering more invasive treatments.

The low back area is unique in its design. The lumbar spine (low back) has the same functions as the rest of the spine, the mid-back and the neck: support, connection, movement, balance, and protection. Yet the low back is designed with a close connection to the pelvis and larger, thicker, and heavier bones than the other bones of the spine. The slight forward curve of the low back counterbalances the slight backward curve of the mid-back. The discs of the low back, made up of fibrous rings that surround an inner gel-like center with layers of fibrocartilage, are thicker than the discs above. The design of the bones and discs of the low back allows for forward, backward, and side bending movement, but rotation is limited due to this design. The discs provide surfaces for the shock-absorbing inner gel. If the bones and discs in the low back area are misaligned or out of balance, low back pain is often the result.

Deep Back Line guidewires are designed to support the low back and pelvis beautifully. On each side of the base of the spine there are two joints, called the sacroiliac joints, made up of strong ligaments that connect the sacrum to the ilium of the pelvis. These deep sacral fascial fibers provide strength and stability. As foundation joints, they are essential for low back support.

Right above these foundation joints are the semi-foundation joints and the myofascia of the low back. The semi-foundation joints are made up of ligaments and cartilage that connect each lumbar vertebra to the other all the way up to the thoracic and neck vertebrae. The myofascial guidewires connect the whole spine, from low back

---

46 Foreman, Judy. (2014). *A Nation in Pain.* New York, Oxford University Press, p. 229.

up to the back of the neck, elegantly. This group of myofascia in the deep low back and above is called the transversospinalis muscle group. This area is where the slow-twitch fibers of the deep inner core provide you with the support you need to align, balance, and move with ease. Freeing these areas and rehydrating the fascia here affects the whole body, from the inside out and from feet to crown.

(To bring the front and back guidewires together, see the Vertical Core Training exercises in Part 4, Step 10.)

MY SUSTAINABLE BODY STORY: HOLDING PLANK POSE USING THE INNER CORE

Since I developed my method of connecting to the center of gravity and the vertical inner core by lying on a soft foam roller and following a specific sequence, I now start my day with this practice. I make sure to connect to my inner core before my yoga, barre, and boot camp classes. I notice that these classes feel easier than they used to; I am challenged, but I don't strain. At the end of a recent boot camp session, the teacher challenged us to hold plank longer than our usual one or two minutes. She challenged us by announcing the record in the former classes that day was five minutes and ten seconds. I joined my fellow boot campers in trying to meet the challenge. As I held my plank longer than the usual two minutes, I focused on my center of gravity and inner core muscles. Slowly, people in the class started to drop out. I kept going. Soon another woman—a marathon runner and athlete—and I were the only ones left. My teacher commented on my alignment. I stayed with my inner core connections and beat the record: five minutes and thirty seconds. I knew I could do this because I engaged my inner core! I had just turned sixty-four and could hold plank longer than many in the class who were half my age. I was proud of myself!

To Sum Up: The Vertical Core

It is good to strengthen your abdominal, gluteal, and back muscles. It is good to do plank holds and yoga poses. Yet it is essential to know about the deep inner Vertical Core that runs from the arches of your feet to the top of your spine, to reconnect to it as a whole, and to train it well. Since these guidewires are what your body uses to stabilize itself, training them frees up your movement muscles from attempting to hold you up. Since these guidewires register your deeper chronic tensions and gripping patterns without you realizing it, training them allows those deeper tension and gripping patterns to release. And since these guidewires allow you to negotiate between moving and holding still in relationship to gravity, training them enables your posture to be effortless.

When these fascial guidewires are not connected and in balance, you lose connection to your body's architecture, which is designed to align, support, and balance you. This is the perfect storm for chronic pain to develop. By treating and training these guidewires, you will be empowered to relieve your pain from the inside out. See Part 4 to learn how to connect to these guidewires.

CHAPTER 11

TRAUMA AND THE VERTICAL CORE

To sustain a healthy life, the body depends on the sympathetic nervous system (arousal) and parasympathetic nervous system (calming) to work with each other in equilibrium. You need the sympathetic nervous system to be aroused when you experience good stress as well as external threats, whether real or perceived. You need the parasympathetic nervous system to balance you for relaxation, sleep, rest, replenishment, and nourishment. When stress is great, and the threat is present, the sympathetic nervous system goes into a fight-or-flight response, where you either stand your ground and fight, or you run to resolve the stress. Once the stress or threat has passed, the parasympathetic nervous system kicks in in order to balance the aroused sympathetic nervous system. The seesaw back and forth keeps you out of perpetual stress and allows your body to replenish itself.

The Vagus Nerve and the Freeze Response

There is another response to stress or to a threat that does not involve fight or flight. It is called the freeze response, and it has unique effects in the body. Several leaders in the field are focusing on the importance of understanding how to work with the effects of trauma as it shows up in the nervous system. The Polyvagal Theory, introduced by Dr. Stephen Porges, emeritus professor of the Brain Body Center at the University of Illinois at Chicago, looks specifically at the role of the vagus nerve, one of the largest nerves in the body.[47] There are two functionally distinct branches of the vagus, or tenth cranial, nerve. The dorsal, or back, branch is the most primitive. It begins at the base of the brain, travels down along the spine, wraps around the heart and lungs, and

---

47 Carter, S. and Porges, Stephen. 2013. *Evolution, Early Experience and Human Development.* New York, NY: Oxford University Press.

descends into the digestive tract into the stomach. The dorsal vagus nerve integrates information from the gut, heart, and lungs. The ventral, or front, vagus nerve, controls the muscles of the face, heart, and lungs, as well as the more rational parts of our brain.[48]

Because of Porges's research, we now know that the vagus nerve is a major part of the parasympathetic nervous system. The vagus nerve brings the neurological and biochemical processes together to regulate our response and recovery from traumatic events. Normally, the dorsal vagus nerve helps keep us in balance between arousal and relaxation. However, when the stress response is too strong, the dorsal vagus nerve can shut down the entire system. The sympathetic nervous system, which normally regulates our fight-or-flight response to stress, becomes so overstimulated that the body cannot handle the signals. The body responds by shifting into the parasympathetic nervous system, where the vagus nerve communicates to the body's systems. We "freeze" in response to the stress.

When we experience trauma or shame (developmental trauma), the vagus nerve is involved. Humans and animals have different ways of responding to this kind of stress and trauma. When an animal "freezes," it may play dead. When the threat is gone, the animal "reawakens," shakes to discharge the freeze response, and goes on its way. In humans, we often do not discharge the nervous system by shaking. This can have a long-term effect on the nervous system. If the freeze response is not discharged from our bodies, many physical and emotional symptoms can result.[49] If we do not discharge and reregulate the nervous system after a stressful or traumatic event, an imprint in the body can set up states of reactivity and disconnection. These are the patterns that become stuck in the fascia, contributing to physical and emotional pain.

As we discussed previously, the communication between the sympathetic and the parasympathetic nervous systems is going on through the sensory nerves in the neurofascial system. We have also covered how the Vertical Core, because it is located

---

48 The ventral (front) vagus nerve is more recent in our evolution. It is called the social engagement nerve because it can determine our expression and responses to other people and how we respond or perceive threats. This nerve allows us to respond to threats in a more tempered way.

49 Lyon, Bret. (2012 Jan 14). Anatomy of a Freeze - or Dorsal Vagal Shutdown. Retrieved from http://eiriu-eolas.org/2012/01/17/anatomy-of-a-freeze-or-dorsal-vagal-shutdown/

deep in the body and close to important bones and joints, is intimately connected to the autonomic nervous system. Remember where the Deep Front Line and Deep Back Line are located. It is my belief that the sensory nerves in the fascia of the Vertical Core tend to hold the body's reactions to stress and trauma: fight, flight, or freeze (see Chapter 7). These reactions become neurological patterns stored deep within the fascia under our conscious awareness. How these patterns are stored and how to release them may be important for lasting healing from trauma.

Holding Patterns in the Vertical Core: My Story

I was a sensitive little girl. My family appeared to others as happy and loving—we were a model of the 1950–1960s perfect *Leave It to Beaver* nuclear family. Yet, when others were not around, it was a different picture. What looked perfect on the outside, was not so perfect inside. When there were no other witnesses, and my father had been drinking, he would explode in anger. Family life seesawed between happy and perfect to loud and angry. Family dinners alternated between pleasant conversation and loud altercations. This seesaw of tensions became the fabric of my life growing up. Little did I know that my body was learning to freeze to protect myself from the onslaught. My body began to take on a shape, an emotional shape, as a reaction to the unsafe environment around me.

I am reminded of a passage from Alice Munro's book of short stories, *Hateship, Friendship, Courtship, Loveship, Marriage*. Munro was the 2013 recipient of the Nobel Prize in Literature. She so elegantly writes: "Slowly, a slight physical collapse, a sort of folding, was occurring inside of me without me knowing it. It was [as] if I were an extension ruler and my ankles, knees, hips, and spine were all being brought together at closer angles."

At age ten, when I went to sleepaway camp and was separated from my mother for the first time, I developed asthma symptoms. The symptoms were treated successfully, but I carried this slight physical collapse because of a stifled breathing pattern into my adult life without being aware of it. I was highly functional. I graduated from the top high school in the nation, went to a reputable New England women's college, lived and worked in Australia, traveled around the world alone, and landed a job as an editor at a reputable Boston publishing house. My life was "successful." Little did I know this childhood traumatic imprint remained embedded within my fascial web and the bones floating within it.

Many years later, after these experiences, I was a bodyworker practicing Zero Balancing and Fascial Release as well as practicing Iyengar Yoga daily. I had done a lot of work to balance my bones, release my fascia, and align myself. On one particular day I was doing a Zero Balancing exchange with my teacher and mentor, Jim McCormick (protégé of Fritz Smith and a brilliant practitioner, mentor, and friend). I was experiencing tension in my marriage, tension that had been growing over many years. Except for my close friends and family, few people knew that what looked like a good marriage on the outside was dysfunctional on the inside. My husband was an alcoholic, and I found myself experiencing the same tension of my childhood. But I did not realize how deep this tension went. When I shared with Jim that my marriage was not going well, and I felt shame, he simply listened; he did not judge. This is where the relationship between two people in the giving and receiving of hands-on work is key: how safe do you feel? I felt safe with Jim.

As the Zero Balancing session unfolded, I was able to sink into Jim's hands and trust that he could hold and support me in the ways I needed. In this session, the shift into feeling that I could let Jim support me took time. I did not let go easily, yet I trusted him. It also required Jim's insightful wisdom as a healer on how best to work with me using gentle, supportive words, such as "You are safe," or "I am here." (If words are used well, they can act as verbal fulcrums, supporting a person in addressing their deeper core fears.)

Jim followed the Zero Balancing protocol of working the lower body first—the foundation and semi-foundation joints of the sacrum, low back, pelvis, hips, and feet. The lower body sets the foundation for the upper body. Now that I understand the architecture of the soft tissue skeleton (the Deep Back and Deep Front Lines), I see how intimately connected the bones and fascia along these myofascial meridians are. Once the foundation in the lower body was laid, Jim followed the protocol and moved to the upper body.

As Jim continued to use the conscious touch, as a well-trained Zero Balancer does, to place gentle fulcrums with his hands into the semi-foundation joints along the Deep Back Line fascial guidewires, my body began to relax more deeply. I didn't know it then, but I now believe that the interoceptive sensory nerve endings in the ligaments and joints in the ribs were activated from deep within. Jim placed a fulcrum of support into my left lower rib. Suddenly, a deep well of grief bubbled up inside me. What had been held in the bones and ligaments of that joint was awakened and able to move. With this movement available, my neurofascial system was flooded with information. As this information that was stored in the tissue memory of my inner core surfaced, tears came to my eyes. With the sensory nervous system flooded with this information that had been stuck for years, the tears turned to sobs that I could not control. From the fascial layers deep within my ligaments and bones of my ribs, I released a long-held tissue memory in the deep inner core of bones and fascia.

Jim held the space beautifully as I released this long-held grief. I wondered if this was grief from my early childhood that had been deeply embedded in my bones. But it did not matter if I could analyze or understand. What mattered is that something held deep in my bone memory had been released. I left the session feeling profoundly altered. That fulcrum, in its pure, safe stillness, had opened up possibilities where before there had been none. Then Dr. Smith's theory came into the light: early childhood memories and losses are often held in the bones of the lower rib cage.

I returned home after the session and followed my usual routine with the kids—school pickup, homework, dinner, bath, reading before bed, then bedtime. I came downstairs from the nighttime ritual with my children to see my husband immersed in his nightly routine of watching TV, drinking, and wanting no communication. On this night, I looked at my marriage from a new perspective. The Zero Balancing session had altered a deep energetic and structural core imprint within me. In that moment, I looked at my husband and realized my marriage was over. It was remarkable how clear I felt. A vibrational pattern in the deeper layers of the fascial fabric of the bones had released. It took years to actualize, but the process of separation and then divorce began at that point. It gave me the opportunity to heal this long-held pattern. My journey to live more authentically became possible.

CHAPTER 12

DOMES AND FANS

If we look closely at the myofascial guidewires of the Vertical Core, it is interesting to note that they connect many of the body's joints, from the feet to the jaw. These joints take the shape of domes. A dome is an arch rotated around its central axis. As with arches, the springing of a dome is the point at which the dome rises. The dome-like shape of the bones, ligaments, and tendons in a joint function as the spring-like connections of a biotensegrity structure (see Chapter 6). Arches and domes hold up space, giving us volume and dimension wherever we are in the body. When you imagine the joint's dome-like shape, you bring your attention to how the bones float in a sea of fascial connections. This enhances alignment of that joint and assists the body in absorbing shock.

Dome-shaped joints supported by the four guidewires include the domes of the feet, ankles, knees, hips, roof of the mouth, eye sockets, and the crown of the head. The palm of the hand is also shaped like a dome, even though it is not directly connected to the guidewires. The fascial domes of the pelvic floor (reverse, or bowl-shaped, dome), the diaphragm, and the thorax (top of the rib cage), though not actual joints, form important support structures for the body's inner dimensions. The Vertical Core guidewires connect and align all of these exquisitely designed domes, from the arches of the feet to the crown of the head. When you lose this connection through everyday strain, stress, or injury, you experience pain in one or

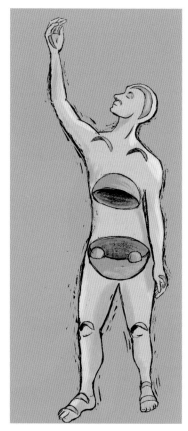

The dome-like architecture of the body, from the feet to the crown. You even have domes in your hands!

more areas—pain that originates from the lack of connection to your inner core support. If your domes are compressed, joint damage ensues. Aligning these myofascial guidewires and the domes along them may be the key to addressing chronic pain issues in the feet, ankles, knees, hips, back, shoulders, neck, and jaw.

By looking at the domes, a whole new body map reveals itself from the inside out. Instead of breaking the body into parts, you can clearly see the body as an integrated architecture with clear connections to the Core Hug and the Vertical Core. The myofascial domes of the body—the pelvic floor, the diaphragm, and the thoracic domes, as well as the roof of the mouth—provide critical support to the body's buoyancy and suspension. By following the step-by-step instructions in Part 4, you can integrate this architecture from arches to crown. This helps you embody the inner relationships of tension, compression, and resilience that are involved in holding you up and keeping you pain-free.

Alignment of each of these domes along the vertical core is critical to whole-body alignment.

In the Sustainable Body Training sequence in Part 4, you will learn how to align your domes and connect them to your inner core. It is important to align the domes of the feet to build a solid foundation for the body. From there you can connect the fascial lines up through the domes of the ankles, knees, and hips, then through the domes of the pelvic floor and diaphragm, and finally up into the roof of the mouth. This will allow you to feel a buoyancy in your architecture that may have escaped your conscious awareness!

Foundation Joints

Joints are where the bones of the skeleton and the ligaments and tendons of the fascial web connect our biotensegrity structures. From the Zero Balancing perspective, some joints ("freely moveable" joints) are mostly used for movement and locomotion, while others—the foundation and semi-foundation joints—are designed to provide stability and transmit forces.[50] Foundation and semi-foundation joints reside in the Deep Front and Deep Back Vertical Core.

---

50 Hamwee, John. 1999. *Zero Balancing: Touching the energy of bone.* London: Frances Lincoln.

The foundation joints include the intertarsal joints that form the dome of the foot, the sacroiliac joints (where the spine connects to the pelvis), the cranial bones of the skull, and the joints that form the dome of the hand. The semi-foundation joints include the small joints that connect the spine to the ribs in the front and the back of the body. What is unique about these joints is:

- they have a small range of motion;
- they are designed to transmit forces;
- we cannot control these joints because they are not under our conscious awareness;
- they hold imbalances rather than resolve them; and
- they cause the body to compensate around them.

They are a major bridge between the energetic and structural core. These joints, I believe, contain many of the sensory nerves of the fascia's interoceptive system, which senses the homeostasis of the body's internal spaces and organs (see Chapter 7). They are also very important to the body's balance and stability.

The Dome of the Foot

Since it is a foundation joint, let's look at the importance of the dome of the foot. If this foundation joint is out of alignment, we cannot align it by an act of will. If we do not get help to realign this kind of joint, it can stay out of place for a long time and the body will start to compensate for the misalignment by manifesting pain somewhere up along the Vertical Core.

Look closely at the five tarsal bones and the ligaments (the springs) between them that form the foundational dome of the foot. This dome-like design allows weight to be carried over a space. As you walk or run, the whole weight of the body comes down on the foot. Without balance and space among the bones and ligaments here, the foot would be crushed on impact. The dome spreads the weight of your body over a space so it can be absorbed through the heel, the ball of the foot and the toes. This absorption of impact through the bones and ligaments of the foot protects the whole body from being compressed into gravity. Our biotensegrity structures can take a lot of force and distribute a force evenly when the bones and ligaments are aligned and hydrated.

If the domes of the feet are not balanced and aligned, the fascial guidewires and major foundation and semi-foundation joints in the spine develop compensation patterns. It was no mistake in the body's vertical design that the guidewires begin in the feet. The feet root us to the earth. A tree's roots grow down into the earth and establish themselves. Just like a tree, our feet must be rooted to the earth to create stability. That stability and grounding down enables us to bounce back up. The architecture of the bones and ligaments of the feet are key to our movement and the transmission of forces. The root system needs to be strong to grow an aligned plant or tree. The domes of the feet need to be aligned and responsive to grow an aligned body.

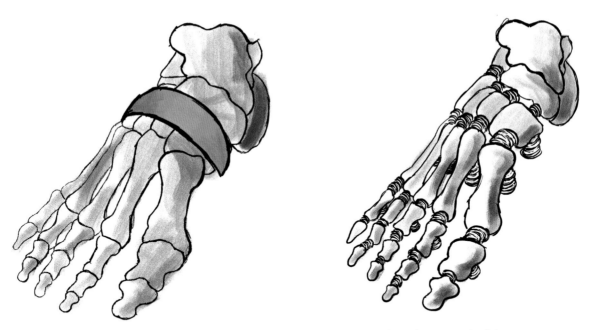

The bones of the feet form a dome (left) and the ligaments between the bones form the springs (right).

TRY IT! MELTING DOMES INTO
THE ARCHES OF THE FEET

In Part 4, you will begin the movement routine by realigning the arches of the feet using a simple, yet profound, process. All you will need is a tennis ball to get started. You will be amazed at the difference you already feel! Erin, one of my clients, shared, "After the first step of tennis ball melting under the foot, I could already feel myself standing more evenly, my spine straightening."

Take a moment and stand with your feet hips-width apart and focus on your feet. If your knees are locked, soften them out of the locked position. What do the arches feel like? Where do you bear weight, on the heels, the balls of the feet, the inner arch or the outer arch? Does your foot have a high arch or a low arch? Now, take a tennis ball or a soft, dome-like object and place it under your arch. Sink down into the tennis ball until you feel a place of resistance. Not too much or too little, but a "hurts good" sensation. Wait until you feel a shift in the sensation. Do not roll the ball around under the foot, just sink into an area and wait until the fascia melts (this can take from ninety seconds to several minutes) Move the ball around to other parts of the arch until the sensations get a little easier. Now, remove the ball from under your foot and feel the space of your arch. Do you notice the difference? You have just created the spatial architecture in your dome. Make sure to do the same with the other foot, so you are balanced. (For full instructions, turn to Part 4, Steps 1 and 2.)

From the Feet Up

Compensation patterns that develop when there is misalignment in the foot dome can be treated from the foot up. Symptoms felt in your knees, hips, abdomen, and upwards are resolved when the whole inner core and the domes within it are addressed. Once the arches of the feet are more balanced, your guidewires can communicate up through the rest of your body more efficiently.

A case that illustrates this is Linda, who came to me complaining of pain in her right knee. She had seen an orthopedist who was recommending surgery to repair a torn meniscus. Upon evaluation of Linda's whole structure, I could see and feel that in addition to her right knee, her right foot and right hip were also out of alignment. She had also manifested sciatica in her right hip in the past. As we worked to balance her foot, ankle, knee, and hip domes, we were able to line up her domes and reconnect the myofascial guidewires. To get the guidewires back in line, Linda worked with creating a balance in the dome of her foot. She then did movement exercises that activated the Vertical Core from the arches of the feet up to her center of gravity, the Core Hug. Her right knee lined up well enough to prevent the need for surgery.

In Western society, people's hips are often tight. Sitting for long hours slumped over the computer or behind the wheel of the car can cause the front guidewires to lock into a shortened position and the back guidewires to lock into a lengthened position, trying to hold up the whole body. The guidewires in the front often need to be treated and restored in their length and lift to relieve the back guidewires and the movement muscles from doing all the postural work.

MY SUSTAINABLE BODY STORY: DEBORAH R.

"I began seeing Karen for help with hip discomfort that developed about four years ago. My right buttock muscles became sore, and over time I could not put much weight on it [when] going up and down stairs. Karen helped identify the true source of the problem, which was sitting with my right leg tucked under me on a very soft swivel chair that I used for work. I never experienced any discomfort in the position, but my hip and buttock muscles, as well as my core, were very much affected. Along with physical therapy, I worked with Karen over the course of the next two years primarily strengthening my core and reactivating muscle groups that had ceased firing properly. My hip pain was relieved."

Disconnection from the Core

Diane had several major surgeries during her lifetime: two cesarean surgeries, her appendix was removed, and she had a partial and then a full hysterectomy. In addition, she had a tummy tuck. Diane is an example of how the connection to the Core Hug and the deep Vertical Core can be severed due to surgery. The pelvic and diaphragmatic domes could not connect to create the tone and suspension the body needs to hold itself up. The connection to the vital psoas muscle was lost (see Chapter 10), and her neurofascial connections were compromised.

As a result, Diane had chronic tension in her neck and shoulders, and her breathing was shallow. Her internal organs needed space and release so her neurofascial system could be more balanced. Using the methods you will learn in Part 4, Diane was able to regain connection to her Vertical Core and Core Hug and thus her pelvic and diaphragmatic domes from within. With this course of treatment, Diane's chronic neck and shoulder pain subsided.

Fans and Triangles

In addition to the body's domes, myofascial fans and triangles are another important architectural component that supports alignment in the body.[51] Yes, we have myofascial fans (muscles and fascia) in our bodies that have a similar shape to handheld paper fans. The handles of the fans begin at a joint structure and open and widen out as they expand through the fascial weave. They are shaped like a slice of a pie. This shape

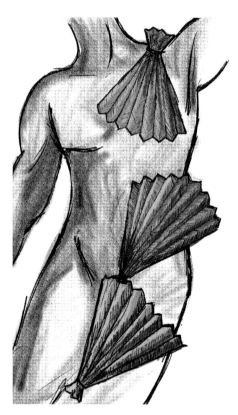

Fans form a structural support of lift and width.

51 Myers, Thomas. 2014. *Anatomy Trains: Myofascial Meridians for Manual and Movement Therapists, 3rd Edition.* Churchill Livingstone.

supports and suspends places in the body. If you look at the actual direction of muscle fibers, they are all in this fan shape.

Just as we examined domes, looking at fans in relationship to the Vertical Core gives us a whole new map of the body. You have fans in your inner thighs, hips, and shoulders. The inner thigh and hip fans are part of the Vertical Core. The shoulder fans suspend off the Vertical Core guidewires and the inner domes. These myofascial fans add width and dimension to your architecture. They support and suspend your domes, especially in the pelvis. When your fans are closed up and stuck, your structure collapses

CASE STUDY: INNER THIGH FANS

Paul arrived in my office complaining of chronic back and left hip pain that had been going on for more than thirty years. He had just learned to live with it. His structure was compromised from being bowlegged and had to negotiate gravity under more extreme compensation patterns. Paul had played basketball all through high school and college. All that jumping required his body to work with gravity from a disadvantaged position. His inner thigh fans were closed down, weak, and disconnected. His hip and back were compensating for the lack of space and support the inner thigh fans should provide to the pelvis and spine. Even though he worked out every day, there was no change in the pain.

We worked diligently with opening the inner thigh and hip fans and balancing the pelvis from the inner Vertical Core guidewires. Paul's knees also felt the brunt of the collapse of the inner thigh fan and inner arch. As I worked the vertical guidewires and widened the inner thigh and hip fans from there, aligned the domes of the feet and the knees, Paul noticed increased ability to buoy his knee, hip and spine up out of gravity.

With regular treatments of the Vertical Core guidewires and the widening of the fans from there, Paul was finally able to feel some length, space, and ease in his hip and spine. He practices the movement routine regularly to sustain the alignment created during the sessions.

into gravity and cannot rebound as efficiently. By opening and widening these fans with the support of the Vertical Core guidewires, you are more buoyant and better able to sustain alignment.

You will learn how to open up your inner thigh, hip, and shoulder fans in Part 4, steps 8, 9, 13, and 14.

Triangles

If we look at the back of the body, the myofascia is designed in the shape of inverted triangles, rather than pie slice-shaped fans. All your back muscles are in the shape of inverted triangles that come to a point at the base of the spine. The front myofascial fans are designed to be widened, lifted, and expanded to open up the front body. The back triangles respond to this opening in the front by relaxing and releasing down the back. Through the connection to the center of gravity and the Vertical Core guidewires, the fans can be opened, lifted, and hydrated in the front body. With this connection, the body's back triangles can sink down and rest back into alignment. The shoulder girdle is suspended on the pelvic girdle more effortlessly. All that chronic neck and shoulder pain many of us experience can be treated more effectively. Relying on the seamless vibrational communication through the Vertical Core, the brilliance of our architecture can unfold.

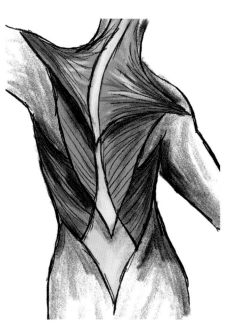

The body's back triangles balancing with the body's front fans.

By following the step-by-step instructions in Part 4, you will integrate the fans and triangles that reside in your body's brilliant architecture.

Building a foundation first

An effective way to treat chronic neck and shoulder pain is to create foundational support in the lower body. The lower body needs to connect into the earth and take that connection through the vertical fascial guidewires into the upper body. This allows the neck and shoulders to rest on the lower body for support. If we are not connected to the Core Hug and Vertical Core, this support cannot happen. The upper body will go into overdrive trying to hold itself up. There is no resting place, so the movement muscles grip, trying to create a foundation of support. The inner core tightens, and the upper body is in perpetual holding.

CASE STUDY: SHOULDER FANS AND BACK TRIANGLES

When Fran complained of constant upper back and neck pain with tingling down her arms and a history of frozen shoulder, I knew we had to help her body connect to her foundation. Her pectoral fans were closed down and folded in. She was hunching over her computer, her camera, and her garden.

Fran connected to her foundational support and brought that support up into her upper body through the Vertical Core and Core Hug. Using touch, I melted the fascial fabric of the shoulder fans at the front of her shoulders and brought the back triangles down the back to align the whole shoulder girdle. Fran began to sense the buoyancy within her fascia that gave her ease and a sense of lift. Her upper back and neck began to relax from the deep Vertical Core of support. Her shoulder fans could melt open, and her back triangles could relax down when they felt support from below. Eventually, her upper back and neck strain melted out of the fascial net. She began to sense how she could suspend her shoulders, neck, and head without straining. Upright posture became a possibility. Lying on the roller reset her connection so that she did not fall back into the old patterns of holding.

To Sum Up: Domes and Fans

In the Sustainable Body Training sequence, you will learn how to align your domes and connect them to your inner core. It is important to align the domes of the feet to build a solid foundation for the body. From there you can connect the fascial lines up through the domes of the ankles, knees, and hips, then through the domes of the pelvic floor and diaphragm, and finally up into the roof of the mouth. You will learn how to open and stretch important myofascial fans of the body (and their back body counterpart, triangles) that often get closed down and stuck, which causes chronic pain. Once these myofascial fans are open, you will reconnect them to the center of gravity and the Vertical Core. By becoming aware of your domes, fans, and triangles, you will be one step closer to relieving chronic pain.

Summing Up Your Body's Brilliant Design

In Part 2, you have learned that the body organizes itself around a point, the Core Hug, and a line, the Vertical Core. When you reconnect to this internal infrastructure through breath and subtle movement, you begin to use your body more efficiently. The subtle sensations emanating through the sensory nerves, especially the slow-twitch fibers of the inner core, help you to feel these connections and use them to move out of pain. As you embody the deep architecture from within, the domes of your joints and myofascial core rebalance. This supportive balance allows your myofascial fans to open wide and the myofascial triangles in the back to sink into a resting position. This new imagery of fascia gives you a chance to envision what is happening in your body, so you can use it to align yourself from the inside out. Understanding your body from this paradigm of support and movement is a huge shift from the Muscle Man concept of levers and pulleys of mechanical movement. Embodying your fascial weave from the inside out may lead to new avenues for treating your long-standing chronic pain issues.

Chronic pain can be alleviated if you realign, repair, rehydrate, and restore these fascial guidewires and the important joints and bones to which they connect. How do you realign and reconnect these guidewires within the fascial web to achieve effortless sitting, standing, and walking in everyday life? The answer lies in how you breathe and the movements you make.

PART THREE

BREATH AND MOVEMENT

"Bask in the brilliance of your body's design."

—Phil Earnhardt

CHAPTER 13

IN CONSTANT MOTION

"The unifying weave of fascia carries and distributes the impulse to move. . . . Fascial initiation is a more holistic experience than what the more differentiated muscles feel. It is impossible to move through the fascia without feeling it transferring and undulating its forces through the entire body. . . . It is a fluid sensation—like noticing a current in the ocean that was already there, and allowing it to express itself into a larger movement."[52]

Breathing: Constant Movement

Since you are not designed for static structural stability, your body is always in motion. Even when you are still, you are moving. When you breathe, you are moving. Yes, it is subtle movement, but it is key to freeing chronic pain. Remember when you were practicing the Core Hug breath in Chapter 9? You started the breath deep in your soft belly and it flowed up naturally into your upper chest. As you breathe in, the dome of the diaphragm goes down to meet the reverse dome of the pelvic floor. This movement touches all the organs in between. As you breathe out, the diaphragm rises up toward the heart and lungs. This up and down movement of the dome of the diaphragm nourishes all the organs, which are enveloped in their fascial sacs. Anatomically, the pelvic floor muscles and the diaphragm together form a supportive spaciousness within your inner core. Your breathing creates movement, which also touches your heart as it beats continually. Your organs relish this up and down movement and use it to digest and process your food.

There is no time you are without movement, except at death. This is why slow, deep belly breathing is so fundamental to your health and well-being. Unfortunately, we

---

52 Townsend, Patty. 2016 Jul 14. Embodied Tensegrity, Fascia, and Yoga. Embodyogablog.com. Retrieved from https://embodyogablog.com/2016/07/14/embodied-tensegrity-fascia-and-yoga/

believe we have to suck in our stomachs or force the pelvis into a tilt. This gripping of your muscles blocks the communication needed for the fascia to communicate to all the different organs and parts of your body. It is important to reconnect to soft belly breathing so you can move through the fascial web seamlessly. Breathing releases the tension and stuck fascia around the organs. In this way, breath can be a profound tool for releasing chronic pain.

Movement: The Latest Findings in Neuroscience and Psychology

Just as deep belly breathing is a profound tool for dealing with chronic pain, so is multi-dimensional movement. Even the academic community is catching up to the fascial scientists in this department. Guy Claxton, a professor of the learning sciences and one of the leading thinkers on creativity, education, and the mind, draws on the latest findings in neuroscience and psychology to affirm what fascia researchers have already discovered: our bodies are in constant motion with a complex communication system.

In his latest book, *Intelligence in the Flesh*, Claxton discusses embodied intelligence as one of the most exciting areas of contemporary philosophy and neuropsychology today. Claxton reiterates what those of us working in the fascia and movement fields have known: the body communicates as a whole system. The name he gives to this concept is Complex Adaptive Dynamic Systems, or CADS for short.[53] As we have discussed, this whole system is made possible by fascia, with its deeply integrated neurofascial communication system. The fascial system communicates throughout the body: from head to toe, from skin to bone, from cell to cell, from organ to organ.

Claxton goes on to say that the system may look reasonably stable, but this kind of solidity is maintained only through constant dynamic movement. This movement is exactly what we refer to when we talk about the fascial web, the neurofascial system, and biotensegrity.

---

53 Friston (2010) as cited in: Claxton, Guy. (2015). *Intelligence in the Flesh: Why your mind needs your body much more than it thinks*. Yale University Press.

Claxton's theory states that every part of our body responds to the other parts. Your body is in constant vital interaction. You are like whirlpools and eddies in a river. You are like clouds and waves. You are like spinning tops that have stability, actively resisting being knocked off course only because you are constantly being spun. "The coherence of bodily structure and behavior reflects the constant internal resonance of all the ingredients with each other—and with the wider set of systems within which they are embedded."[54]

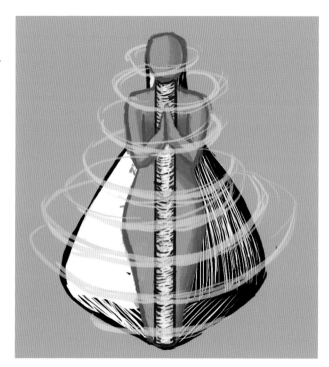

After reading this passage, an image came to me: I saw the body as a constantly spinning top. The center of gravity (the Core Hug) in the pelvis was in the lower and thicker base of the top. The myofascial guidewires of our Vertical Core are how the top (your body) is constantly being spun but does not topple over because it is where the coherence of the bodily structure resides. It is only through movement, or the "constant internal resonance of all the ingredients with each other,"[55] that we find our balance and alignment.

You are a dynamic system orienting around a point and a line.

54 Claxton, Guy. (2015). *Intelligence in the Flesh: Why your mind needs your body much more than it thinks.* Yale University Press.

55 Claxton, Guy. (2015). *Intelligence in the Flesh: Why your mind needs your body much more than it thinks.* Yale University Press.

CHAPTER 14

FUNCTIONAL MOVEMENT

To harness the power of movement and combat a sedentary lifestyle leading to chronic pain, many of us turn to exercise. What is important is not the exercise that you do, but rather how aligned you are when doing it. Many issues of chronic pain come from people living sedentary lifestyles in poor alignment, and then doing exercises too quickly and too vigorously.

Poor Exercise Habits and a Sedentary Lifestyle

Repetitive exercise, particularly if the exercise is done in misalignment, can have negative effects on the fascia. Fascial scientists discovered that repetitive movement dehydrates the fascia; it gets stuck. Do you spend many hours of the day sitting in front of a computer, driving a car, or hunching over handheld devices? When you stay in the same position for hours and do not move, you are drying out your fascia. And if you sit with poor posture, rounded back and shoulders, you easily disconnect from your inner core, which needs to be used to lengthen your spine and align your shoulders and neck on top of it. Do you then seek exercise and fitness routines to counteract all those hours of not moving? Are you aware of how to place or position your body well before you exercise? If you do not align your body using the inner core before you exercise, you may be doing more harm than good and perpetuating poor postural habits.

When you are connected and aligned from the inner core, you're using your body the way it was meant to be used. When you are not aligned in this way, you're likely using the muscles designed for movement, instead of the muscles designed for posture. Since the movement muscles are not designed to support alignment in the way postural muscles are, you're overusing them, and they let you know by sending you messages of tightness, soreness, and pain. If you exercise without training your inner core and using its support for alignment, you may aggravate your pain.

If you follow a traditional weight lifting program or a fitness training, you tend to concentrate on one muscle group. For example, you do bicep curls that isolate and strengthen the anterior bicep muscles. When you use machines at the gym to strengthen specific muscles, you're training those muscles in mechanical ways. Unfortunately, these exercises that isolate muscle groups do not necessarily help you use the muscles the same way you would in your day-to-day movements. When you reach to grab a ball, you are not only using the anterior biceps, you use a whole array of muscles in the arm, shoulder, neck, back, and lower body. How muscles are used in coordinated and fluid ways is determined by your fascia, because all muscles are connected by fascia. Most every movement you make in life involves the whole body and the whole fascial system. That is why it's so important to train the fascia as a whole system rather than isolated parts. By micromanaging the variables acting on the individual muscles, you lose the unifying, undulating forces throughout the whole body. When this dynamic way of moving is lost, chronic pain can be a result.

Functional Movement

How you move in everyday life affects how you are living in your fascia. A term that describes this concept is "functional movement." Functional movements are the movements we do repeatedly on a daily basis. Our fascia makes functional movements possible, so making sure your fascia is fit is important in more ways than we knew.

Picture this:

A young student in yoga class performs the poses in perfect alignment, but once class is over, she takes out her cell phone and immediately rounds her back and hunches over to look at it. She walks out of the class in this posture. This describes her functional movement. She may have chronic pain no matter how many yoga classes she attends.

A professional dancer whose body is perfectly aligned moves with easy grace when she performs. Yet when she cuts vegetables in the kitchen, she rounds her shoulders and hunches over the counter. Even though she is aligned while she dances, her fascia takes on the shape of her rounded shoulders. She may experience chronic pain in her shoulders and neck.

In fitness class, students go through the exercises, but their bodies are in poor alignment while doing them. The students leave class stronger in certain muscle groups, but weaker in others. Fitness class may not relieve their chronic pain; it may even exacerbate it.

A web designer, who sits for hours at the computer in poor posture, goes to yoga classes to counteract the stresses of work and ends up with tendinitis in his elbow because he continued to round his shoulders as he performed yoga poses.

In all the above examples, I ask each individual this question: how do you sit, stand, and walk in everyday life? Functional movement is posture in motion, so how about using your center of gravity and the fascial Vertical Core guidewires to guide your posture in motion. If you use the body's brilliant design to balance and align yourself in everyday movement, poor posture, stuck fascia, stuck stress, and poor movement patterns can be addressed. Maybe you can join those in cultural lifestyles where sitting, standing, and walking in the architecture of the body has not been lost.[56] If you sit, stand, and walk using your architecture well, these movements squeeze and release the stuck fascia and allow the bound tissues to refill with the juicy fluids of the fascia.[57] Imagine you are sitting, standing, and walking with a distinct ease and fluidity, using your fascial architecture so well that chronic pain is a thing of the past.

---

56 An example on YouTube shows how one man uses his body's architecture to carry twenty-two bricks on his head while walking on a narrow plank. Even though the man is not big and muscular, he is stronger than most. His strength comes from his functional movement, using his center of gravity and his Vertical Core deep within the fascial web. (Go to YouTube and type in "Man with 22 bricks," or visit https://www.youtube.com/watch?v=uc_We9WXxSI, to enjoy watching the body's brilliant design in action.)

57 This is the premise behind Fascial Fitness. Fascial Fitness has four components: soft tissue stretching, which moves away from single, one-muscle stretches and into whole-body myofascial chain stretching; rebound elasticity, or training the fascia back into the bouncy elasticity of our "kid body"; fascial release, using a roller to soften fascia and create space; and fluid refinement, which trains our sensory nervous system through our awareness and a variety of movements.

The exercises in Part 4 train the body's inner core so that your functional movement patterns are more stable and fluid. Being aligned from your inner core using your sustainable body allows exercise to be more beneficial—and the strains of daily living are lessened.

CHAPTER 15

CONNECTING ALL THE PARTS USING BREATH AND MOVEMENT

I cannot stress enough how important breath and movement are to the fitness of your fascia, your alignment, balance, and, ultimately, your overall health. Since fascia does not have its own blood supply, breath and multi-vector movement is the only way it can nourish, cleanse, and rehydrate itself. Stuck fascia means stuck stress and chronic pain. We all know exercise is helpful, but what kind of exercise and how it is done is also important. Are you overworking some muscles and underworking others? Are you doing your exercises in alignment, or are you stressing your body by doing exercises out of alignment? Are you exercising the outer core and neglecting the inner core? Exercise alone may not be the solution; the way you exercise and how you move when you are not exercising also play roles in alleviating chronic pain. Let me teach you a new way to do this.

Think about how you sit, stand, and walk in your daily life. Simple changes to these movements may be what actually helps alleviate your chronic pain!

1. How do you sit? Are you slumped forward, are you overarching your low back, or are you balanced evenly between the two positions?
2. How do you stand? Do you stand on both legs evenly, or do you tend to sink into one hip and leg?
3. How do you walk? Are you walking with your whole body relaxed, or are you walking only with the legs or only with the head, neck, shoulders, and arms?

How you sit, stand, and walk tells a lot about your posture. You can use breath and movement to change your postural patterns. You will be learning how to do this in the

Sustainable Body Training sequence in Part 4. The exercises, when done with breath and awareness, help you listen to and follow your body's design.

The Big Picture

My premise is simple: there is an architecture within your body that is designed to align, balance, and suspend you. Your body connects to this architecture through a body-wide neurofascial system that communicates head to toe, skin to bone, organ to organ, and cell to cell. If the fascia is stuck and dehydrated because of injury, poor posture, stress, and/or repetitive movement, this neurofascial communication works less efficiently. You can unstick, realign, and rehydrate this neurofascial system from the inside out using breath and movement. Your body is designed with a center of gravity (the Core Hug) that you can connect to using your breath, and a deep inner core (the Vertical Core) that you can connect to using subtle movement while you balance on a soft foam roller.

When you understand how to connect to the center of gravity and the inner core, you can access your alignment, balance, and suspension with relative ease. Using this connection to your body's brilliant design, you can align the domes, fans, and triangles that depend on these deeper inner core connections for support. These connections help you relieve chronic pain, prevent injury, and sit, stand, and walk in the way you were designed to move. Now it's time to learn exactly how you can make these connections to your body's brilliant design.

PART FOUR

SUSTAINABLE BODY TRAINING SEQUENCE

"Movement is a medicine for creating change in a person's physical,

emotional, and mental states."

—Carol Welch

A Note on Mindful Exercise

Because fascia holds your proprioceptive nerves (the nerves that sense position and movement within the body), it important to do the following exercises with mental attention, or a state of mindfulness, for maximum benefit.[58] Studies in the fields of complementary therapies have shown that paying attention to the movements one makes can lead to a reduction in pain. In one study, patients with complex regional pain syndrome experienced significant improvement of their condition when they paid attention to the sensations in their body rather than being mentally distracted (i.e., reading a book) during treatment.[59] Mindful attention was a "prerequisite to gain therapeutic effects."[60]

For the following exercise routine, it is important to pay close attention to the sensations in your body for maximum benefit. You need to repeatedly sense the connections you make to your Core Hug and your Vertical Core so your body can organize around a point and a line. Always use your awareness and breath to initiate each movement. If you go directly into muscular movement, you will simply use your habitual patterns. For this reason, I have included steps that remind you to come back to these sensations and reassess your alignment throughout the routine.

The Soft Foam Roller

The Sustainable Body training sequence involves lying down vertically on a soft foam roller. By placing the whole spine on a soft roller, you are better able to connect to the dimensions of your fascial web and the architecture within you. I highly recommend you invest in a roller for maximum benefit from this program.[61]

---

58 Schleip, Robert (ed.). 2015. *Fascia in Sport and Movement*. East London: Handspring Publishers, p.34.
59 Moseley et al. (2007), as cited in Schleip, Robert (ed.). 2015. *Fascia in Sport and Movement*. East London: Handspring Publishers.
60 Ibid.
61 I recommend OPTP's Pro-Roller™ Soft model, available at www.optp.com.

It is important to use a soft roller for the Sustainable Body training sequence. The soft roller allows the sensory nerve endings in the fascia to receive the correct input from the inner core. Since we are aiming to reconnect your neurofascial system, which is most likely stressed and strained, the body needs to be able to relax. The autonomic nervous system needs to move out of the stress response and into the rest response. Balancing the whole spine on a soft foam roller helps the neurofascial system restore and balance itself from the inside out.

What will you be able to do by using the soft foam roller?

1. The roller will help you improve your body awareness and connect you to the mechanisms and signals the body's fascia uses to balance and align itself.
2. You will connect to the center of gravity of the fascial web using breath.
3. You will activate the deep Vertical Core in both the back body and front body, which stabilizes your spine.
4. You will strengthen the signals of communication through the slow-twitch fibers of the deeper fascial layers.
5. You will be able to differentiate between your inner and outer core.
6. You will stretch deep myofascial fans, which will relax and free tight muscles.
7. You will reset the body's domes to remove misalignment and stress from joints.
8. You will perform simple movements slowly and consciously, which allows you to focus on breathing and move with precision.
9. Your awareness will be challenged to make new connections in order to reset alignment for dynamic movement in walking, sitting, and standing.
10. You will reeducate and reconnect to the body's brilliant design.

Supporting yourself on the roller

I have worked with many clients on and off the roller with low, mid, and upper back pain. It can feel scary to perform new exercises when you have pain, so make sure you use what you need to feel supported while on the roller. This may include:

- Placing a folded towel or small pillow under your head to keep the neck in alignment. You will know your neck is aligned when your chin is neither tilted toward the sky nor tucked into your chest, but parallel to the rest of your spine (see photos in Steps 3 and 4).
- Placing firm pillows, towels, or bolsters under your arms on either side of the roller.

To avoid pain or injury, be sure to *always* get onto and off the roller following the directions in Steps 4 and 11.

Precautions and Contraindications

As with any new exercise regime, check with your physician before starting. These practices are not intended to replace the services of your physician or provide an alternative to any medical treatment. To reduce the risk of injury, please consult with your doctor before beginning this or any exercise program.

Listed below are some precautions and contraindications or reasons why you may *not* want to perform these exercises on the foam roller:

1. Severe scoliosis or S curve of the spine
2. Severe kyphosis or rounding of the upper back
3. Vertigo or dizziness
4. Herniated disk or fractured vertebra
5. A recent fracture or sprain
6. Full weight-bearing restrictions
7. Osteoporosis
8. Problems with dislocating shoulders
9. Rheumatoid arthritis
10. Recent surgery
11. Late-term pregnancy
12. Serious long-term illness

If you have any of the aforementioned conditions, you may want to perform the exercises on the floor (with your doctor's permission) or omit them altogether.

On or off the roller

These exercises are designed so all of them can be performed off the roller and the benefits are still felt. For beginners, I suggest you begin by doing all the exercises *on the floor first*. After a few weeks, once you have mastered the routine, try doing the exercises on the roller.

If you have pain during any of the exercises, stop. Check your position and execution of the move. If there is still pain, do the exercise on the floor or omit it from your program. Listen to your body! The wisdom is within. Trust it.

Remember that the roller exercises will help you make the connections needed to stabilize your spine. *Start slowly, modify by doing the exercises off the roller first until you are strong enough to do them on the roller. Please follow the precautions given so as not to irritate an already existing condition.*

Sustainable Body practice

It is beneficial to do the Sustainable Body training whether on the floor or on the roller as a daily practice. Many find it helpful to think of it as a moving meditation. If daily practice is not possible, doing the routine three or four times a week is also beneficial. If you've had a particularly stressful day or spent time doing a repetitive movement, whether it be sitting, gardening, running, or biking, doing the Sustainable Body routine to realign yourself afterwards is helpful and undoes some of the stresses created by repetitive movements. Many find it helpful to do the routine first thing in the morning to undo the compression that happens during sleep. Others find it helpful to do the routine, especially the breathing segment, before bed. This can reduce the accumulation of stress from the day and also help alleviate sleep disorders. If you do the routine prior to going for a walk or run or to a yoga, Pilates, or fitness class, you are laying the foundation of more optimal alignment prior to activity. In other words, the fundamentals of inner core connection and stabilization are taken into your movements. You will find that daily activities and exercises are easier and more fun because you are better aligned, have more strength, and feel more flexible.

STEP-BY-STEP INSTRUCTIONS

My client, Lauren, said to me, "I woke up stiff and sore today, but I did the exercises on the roller and I feel ten times better! They always help. Your work is so sustainable."

You will need:

- a 36-inch soft foam roller[62] (or a hard foam roller wrapped in a towel, blanket, or yoga mat)
- a folded towel or small pillow for neck support
- a tennis ball (or a similar soft, dome-like object) for foot rolling
- a soft 2-pound Pilates ball, or a 1- or 2-pound weight (for step 7)
- two yoga blocks or Pilates rings (optional, for step 15 only)

Let's begin.

1. Feeling Your Roots

Goals: To sense your body in relation to space and in relation to gravity.
To notice where you bear weight in the feet.

Stand, placing your feet hips-width apart. Soften your knees. Let your tailbone sink down gently. Keep your eyes open and look out, not down. Take a soft, slow, deep breath in and out. Sense your body in relation to the space around you. Now, close your eyes. Breathe slowly and deeply, bringing your awareness inside. If your knees are locked, soften them. Bring your attention to your feet. How do they feel in relation to the ground?

Notice where you bear weight in your feet. Do you tend to sink into the heels, or do you have more weight in the forefoot? Do you tend to roll into the inner arches or out into the outer arches? Is there a difference between your two feet? Notice your pattern without judgement. Now, balance the weight of your body between the heel and ball, inner arch and outer arch of each foot. Imagine the domes of your feet lifted and springy.

---

62 I recommend OPTP's Pro-RollerTM Soft model, available at www.optp.com.

2. Melting Domes into the Arches of the Feet

Goals: To melt the fascia in the arches of the feet to awaken the beginning of the Vertical Core.

To create balance, alignment, and suspension in the foundation joints of the feet.

Materials needed: tennis ball

While standing, place the tennis ball under one foot, just behind the ball of the big toe, and stretch your toes toward the ceiling, then sink slowly into the ball, allowing the foot and toes to soften around the ball. When you feel a place of resistance (a wrinkle in the fascia), wait, breathe, and sink into the ball. Only go to the place of resistance where it "hurts good." Do not roll the ball around on the foot. Stay with the "hurts good" feeling until you feel a shift. This is the fascia melting. Look out into space while you do this. Find the sore places in the arch. Slowly melt the whole arch of the foot on the tennis ball. Keep the knees soft. Imagine you are melting the fascia to create a dome in the arch for suspension. Come off the ball, stand, and feel the difference between your feet. Repeat the same sequence on the other foot. Stand, notice how the domes of your arches are activated.

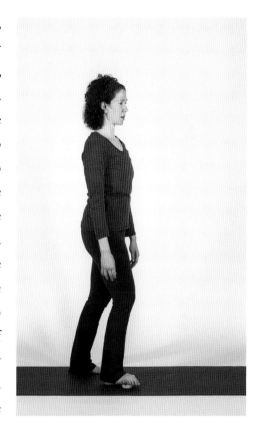

Note: If you have trouble balancing, hold onto a chair or a wall for support while doing this exercise.

3. Assessing Your Alignment

Goal: To use your sensory awareness to feel your body's weights and spaces.

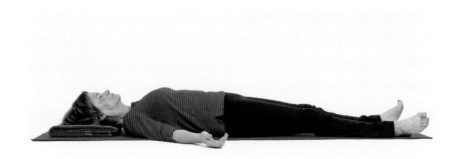

Lie on the floor with your legs straight and relaxed, your arms resting out away from the sides of your body, palms up.

Note: *Make sure your neck is aligned. Place a folded towel or small pillow under your head to support the alignment of the neck. You will know your neck is aligned when your chin is neither tilted toward the sky nor tucked into your chest, but parallel to the rest of your spine (see photo).*

Notice the weights and spaces of your body's architecture. Feel the domes of the feet, the weight of the heels, the space behind the knees, the weight of the pelvis. Feel the space of the low back, the weight of the shoulders, the space in the neck, and the weight of the head. Draw an imaginary line down the middle of your body and notice any differences between the right and left sides. Take a full breath and notice what areas of your body move and those that don't. No judgment, just notice. Take a mental snapshot with your mind's eye of how your body feels in the moment.

Note: *If you are a beginner, start by doing the remaining exercises on the floor first. Once you have mastered the exercises on the floor, move to doing the exercises on the soft foam roller.*

4. Getting into Starting Position

(beginner on floor; intermediate/advanced on roller)

Goal: To get the body into a comfortable position on the floor or the roller.

Materials needed: Foam roller, small folded towel or pillow

Beginner—floor only. Lie on the floor, knees bent, feet hips-width apart, with support of a folded towel under the neck.

Intermediate, advanced—getting onto the roller. Sit up, place your tailbone at one end of the roller with your knees bent, feet flat on the floor about hips-width apart.

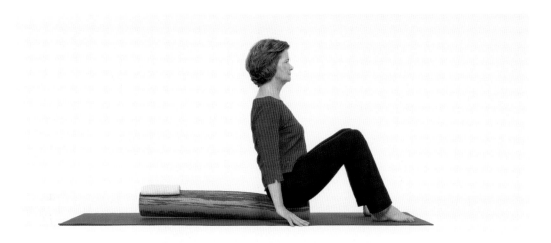

Place your hands on the floor for support and slowly roll yourself down along the length of the roller.

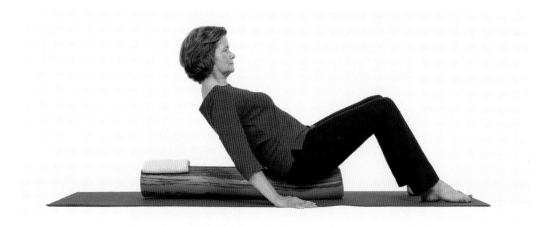

Make sure the spine, from the tailbone to the head, is fully supported on the roller.

Note: *Make sure the neck is aligned with the rest of the spine. To do this, place a folded towel under the head. You will know your neck is aligned when your chin is neither tilted toward the sky nor tucked into your chest, but parallel to the rest of your spine (see photo).*

In order to create space in the spine, gently press your feet into the floor, lift the pelvis, scoop your tailbone down and away from you, then lower your pelvis back down onto the roller. Feel the space in the lower back. Place your hands at the back of your neck, gently lift your head to lengthen your neck, then place your head back down. Feel the length in the neck. Breathe deeply as you sink your spine into the roller. If you have trouble balancing on the roller, place a pillow on each side for support.

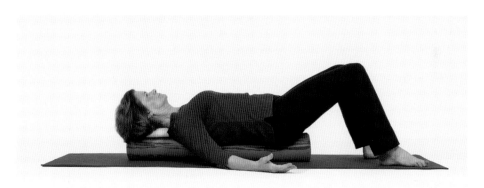

5. Rocking

(beginner on floor; intermediate/advanced on roller)

Goal: To activate the slow-twitch fibers of the Vertical Core.

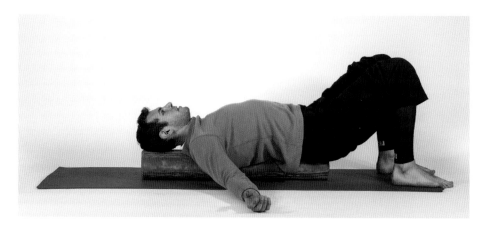

Take a deep inhale. As you exhale, gently rock your whole body to one side, imagining you are a waterfall of molasses slowly pouring into the floor. You want a sense of falling and catching yourself using only your forearm and foot to stop the fall. Allow your whole body to sink into the sense of letting go into the fall, yet simultaneously catching yourself. Breathe slowly and hold for ten to fifteen seconds.

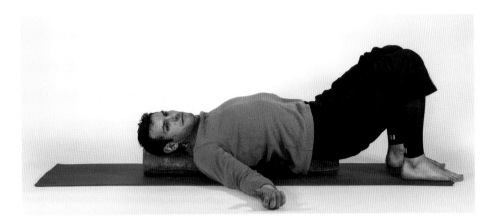

Bring yourself back up into center on the roller (or the floor). Inhale. As you exhale, rock your whole body to the other side. Hold for ten to fifteen seconds. Repeat three to four times, alternating from side to side. Begin each rocking movement with a full inhalation as you lie centered on the roller and with a full exhalation as you rock to the side. Remember to breathe throughout the gentle rocking movements.

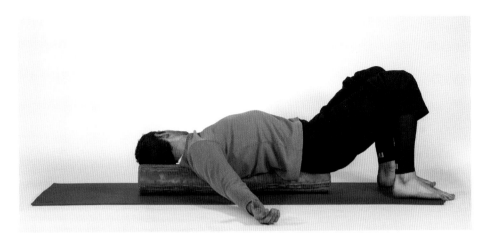

6. Wave Breath

(beginner on floor; intermediate/advanced on roller)

Goals: To activate your breathing muscles and increase pulmonary elasticity.
To align the dome of the diaphragm over the reverse dome of the pelvic floor.
To balance the autonomic nervous system.

Imagine you are at the ocean watching the waves come in and go out. Soften your belly. Take a soft, slow, deep inhalation through the nose. Begin the inhalation deep in your low belly. Imagine your breath is a wave arising out of the ocean of your belly.

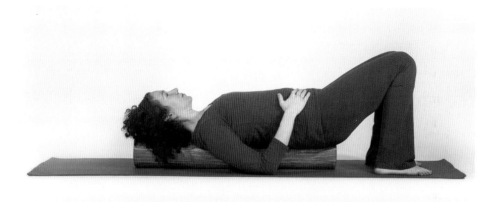

Watch the wave flow up into the collar bones, or the shore of your chest. Pause.

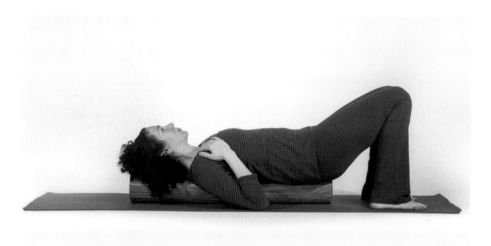

Then, exhale through the nose, softly, slowly, and deeply. Watch the breath like a wave go back into the ocean of your belly. Pause. Watch your breath and match it to the rhythm of the waves. Breath arises out of the ocean of the belly and flows onto the shore of the chest, never forcing or pushing. Notice if you are using your neck or shoulder muscles to bring the breath up onto the shore of your chest. If you are, release these muscles; they are not breathing muscles. Relax them. Inhale and exhale softly, slowly, and deeply through your nose. Repeat four to five times, or until your breath matches the rhythm of the waves.

7. Core Hug Breath

(beginner on floor; intermediate/advanced on roller)
Goals: To use breath to connect to the center of gravity, the single point at the center of the fascial web around which the body organizes.
To bring the muscles and bones of the pelvis together around the center of gravity.
Materials needed: 2-pound Pilates ball or 1- or 2-pound weight

Take a soft, slow, deep inhalation through your nose, noticing the wavelike dimensionality of the breath. On the exhale, softly touch the tip of your tongue to the roof of your mouth and say slowly to yourself, "La, la, la, la," in a soft whisper. *Focus on committing to the end of the exhale.* If you exhale fully, you will sense a slight activation at the center of the body just below the navel and above the pubic bone, this is the Core Hug. Pause. Repeat until you feel the subtle contraction at the end of the exhale.

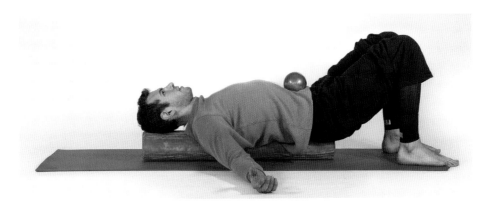

If you do not feel this slight activation, place a soft Pilates ball or a weight just below the navel as a cue for your neurofascial system. This time, as you come to the end of the la-la-la's and you cannot utter one more la, try "lion's breath," sticking out your tongue and blowing out the rest of the air. This maximizes the exhale and allows you to activate the Core Hug more effectively.

If you feel your muscles tensing or gripping, release them. Let the breath do the work, not the muscles. Repeat four to five times.

If the quiet la, la, la exhale breath does not work for you, try counting slowly from one to ten repeatedly, whispering quietly until you reach the end of the exhale.

Now you are ready to connect to the three-dimensionality of the Core Hug:

1) as you come to the end of the exhale and feel the activation in the front belly,
2) gently lift the pelvic floor up toward your navel; and
3) gently press the sacrum, the base of the spine, into the roller (or the floor).

Feel the subtle engagement of your deep center of gravity in its three dimensions. This breathing exercise brings all the bones and muscles of the pelvis together around the body's center of gravity. Let the breath do the work. Let the movements be subtle.

Because of past training, we often make the mistake of thinking we should grip muscles or force the pelvis to tuck. This keeps us out of the neurological connections of the slow-twitch fibers that we need to make to truly feel our inner Core Hug. Keep in mind that a toned belly can be a soft belly. Enjoy giving your core a deep hug. Feel how centered you become.

Rest. Go back to normal breathing. Notice how you can use your awareness to feel the Core Hug with your natural exhale and the connection to the subtle sensations of engagement. This engagement allows you to connect neurologically to the center of gravity. It is not muscular. The sensations are subtle, so go slowly, use awareness, and be patient. **Use this connection to the Core Hug for the rest of the routine.**

8. Melting Inner Thigh Fans

(beginner on floor; intermediate/advanced on roller)

Goals: To melt the fascia of the inner thighs, which forms architectural fans of support. To connect the Vertical Core from the arches of the feet to the Core Hug.

On the roller or the floor, connect to the Core Hug with your natural exhale (step 7), place the soles of your feet together and allow your knees to fall apart toward the floor. Notice your inner thigh fans melting slowly and gently. If the stretch is too much, bring your knees back up, then down slowly, like butterfly wings. To challenge the stretch, rock gently side to side on the roller (or the floor), melting one fan then the other. Place your attention on the subtle sensation of how Core Hug engagement communicates stability to the inner thigh fans.

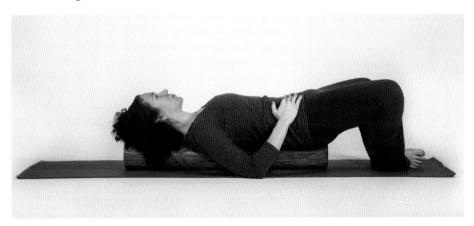

Maintaining the same position with the soles of the feet together, lift just the heels off the floor, pinky toes remain in contact with the floor. Press the big toe mounds and heels together and fan out your toes. As you press, feel the connection from your arches, up the inseam of the legs, and into the Core Hug. Imagine you are tracing the shape of a diamond from your arches into the Core Hug. Repeat four to five times. Return to starting position.

9. Melting Shoulder Fans

(beginner on floor; intermediate/advanced on roller)

Goals: To melt the fascia of the pectoral muscles in front of the shoulders, which forms architectural fans.

To suspend the shoulder joints and align the neck.

To connect the shoulder girdle to the center of gravity and Vertical Core.

On the floor or the roller, connect to the Core Hug (step 7). Reach your arms up over your head into a V, resting the backs of the hands on the floor. If the stretch is too much, bring the arms down to a lower position. The key is to gently melt width into the front of the shoulders. To increase the stretch and hydrate the fascia, rock gently from side to side. Allow your head to rock from side to side to stretch the neck along with the front of the shoulders.

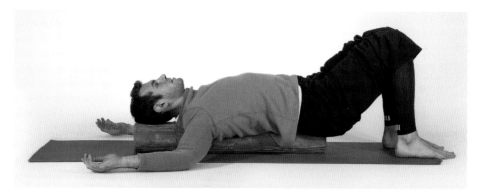

Next, place the palms of the hands together above your head. You may grab one wrist with the other hand and pull gently. Feel the shoulder joints releasing. Alternate between melting shoulder joints and pectoral fans in a way that feels good to you.

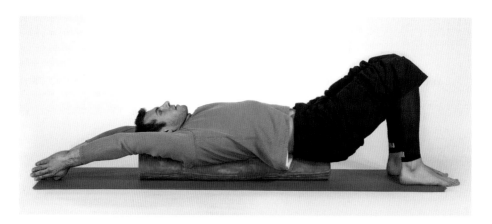

Note: If you have shoulder issues, only go as far as is comfortable. Stop if you feel pain. Work up to melting more space into the shoulders gradually. The shoulder girdle is meant to be suspended on the pelvic girdle, so use this movement to create that suspension.

10. Vertical Core Training

(beginner on floor; intermediate/advanced on roller)

Goals: To activate the slow-twitch fibers of the Vertical Core.

To reconnect to the body's center of gravity and Vertical Core simultaneously.

To go back to the original movements of crawling, standing, and walking in the Vertical Core that we developed as young children.

Two-legged human structures use the center of gravity and the Vertical Core to move with balance and ease. Babies did not have to do sit-ups and planks to be strong enough to sit, stand, and walk. Babies first learn to crawl, then they learn to pull themselves up to standing. Finally, they learn to walk. In this Vertical Core training, you will be going back to those original movements from crawling to walking. This training enables you to reconnect to the balance, stability, and resilience you had as a child.

Beginners: Do all four steps on the floor first. Master each step fully before you progress to the next one. Vertical Core training takes time and focus. If you practice, you will notice a difference in your alignment, balance, and strength. Once you have mastered the movements on the floor, move to the roller. Master each step fully before moving on to the next one.

Intermediate/Advanced: Do all four steps on the roller. For many, these balancing exercises are challenging, as the Core Hug and Vertical Core may have been disconnected for a while. Go slowly and use your full attention. Master Step a before you advance to Step b. Once you have mastered Step b, advance to Step c, and make sure you master it before attempting Step d. Do not assume you will be able to master these movements quickly; it takes time. If you practice, you will notice a difference in your alignment, stability, and strength.

Step a. Baby Crawl

(beginners on floor; intermediate/advanced on roller)

Lie with your knees bent, hips-width apart, arms at your sides. Place a folded towel under your head to align your neck. Connect to your Core Hug (step 7).

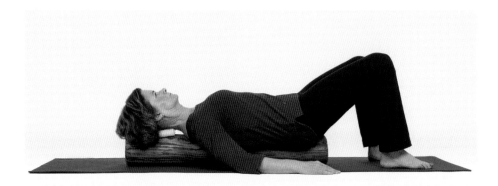

Lift your left leg off the floor, with your knee bent ninety degrees and your foot flexed. Lift your right (opposite) arm off the floor. Place the leg and arm back down.

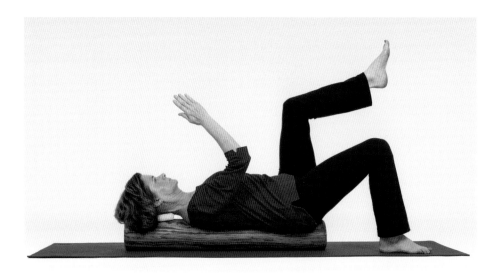

Lift your right leg off the floor, with your knee bent ninety degrees and your foot flexed. Lift your left (opposite) arm off the floor. Place the leg and arm back down.

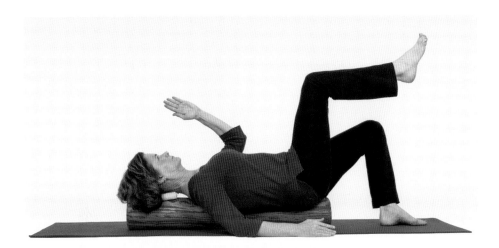

Repeat these moves, lifting opposite leg and opposite arm, six to twelve times. Imagine you are taking a walk. You are making the same movements as you do in crawling.

Note to those on the roller: If you wobble a lot, keep practicing until the connections are made. Do not move on to Step b (Big Kid Crawl) until you are stable on the roller. This may take weeks or even months of practice. That is okay; listen to your body and go at your own pace.

Step b. Big Kid Crawl

(beginners on floor; intermediate/advanced on roller)

With the Core Hug engaged, lift one leg, with the knee bent at ninety degrees and foot flexed, and hold. Lift the other leg, with the knee bent at ninety degrees and foot flexed, and hold. Balance your whole body using the Core Hug. If you are able, straighten one leg up to ceiling, and then lower it back so the knee is bent at ninety degrees. Repeat this motion with the other leg.

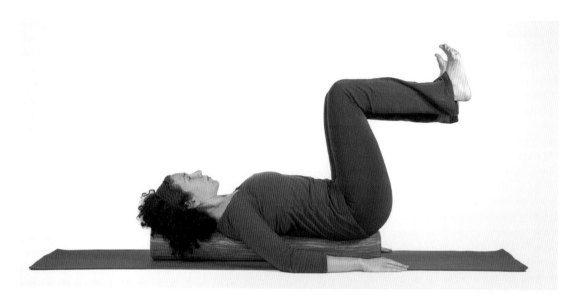

If that is doable, try alternate arm/leg raises from Core Hug. Place your full attention on balancing and moving from the Core Hug.

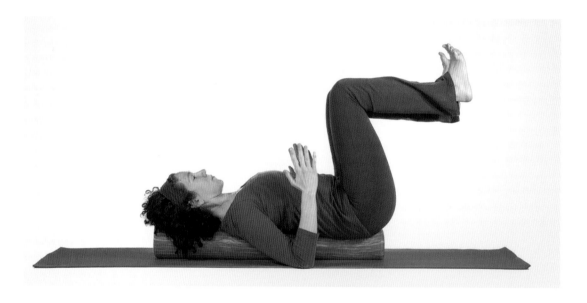

With core hug activated, knees bent ninety degrees, feet flexed: bend both elbows ninety degrees, fingers pointing toward the ceiling.

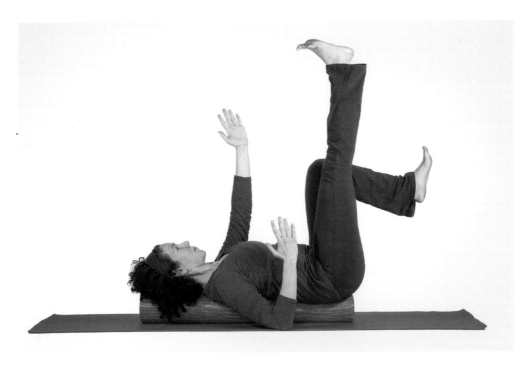

Slowly straighten the right leg, then the left arm toward the ceiling. Hold a few seconds. Return to starting position.

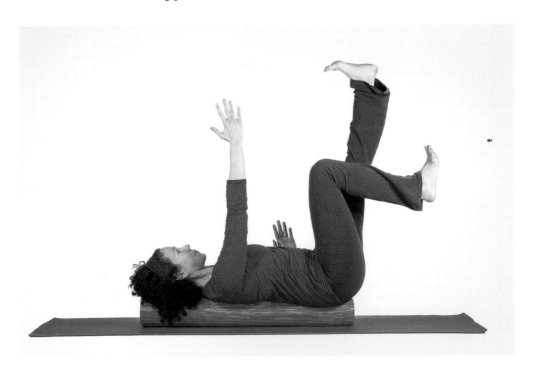

Slowly straighten the left leg, then right arm toward the ceiling. Hold a few seconds. Return to starting position.

Repeat this movement of straightening opposite leg and arm, then return to starting position six to twelve times.

Note to those on the roller: if you wobble a lot, keep practicing until the connections are made. Do not move on to Step c (Standing) until you are stable on the roller. Listen to your body and go at your own pace.

Step c. Standing

(beginners on floor; intermediate/advanced on roller)

With the Core Hug engaged, lift both legs off the floor and straighten them toward the ceiling. Place your arms out to the sides for balance. Very slowly, bring your right leg out to the side about forty-five degrees from the midline. Return your leg to the starting position.

Bring your left leg out to the side about forty-five degrees from the midline. Return your leg to the starting position. Repeat this movement on each side, ensuring that you only bring the leg out forty-five degrees from the center or midline.

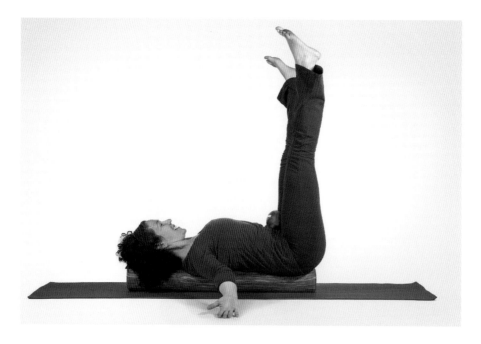

Advanced: With one leg out to the side at a forty-five-degree angle, trace the shape of an oval with the big toe going clockwise. Then counterclockwise. Use the whole leg from the hip to the foot to do this movement. Repeat with the other leg.

Note to those on the roller: if you wobble a lot, keep practicing until the connections are made. Do not move on to Step d (Walking) until you are stable on the roller. Listen to your body and go at your own pace.

Step d. Walking

(beginners on floor; intermediate/advanced on roller)

Note: Each sub-step of the Walking series may be practiced for weeks before moving on to the next step. If you notice yourself losing your connection to the Core Hug, STOP. Keep practicing the previous step until the connections are made. Listen to your body and go at your own pace.

1. With the Core Hug engaged (step 7), lift one leg with your knee bent ninety degrees, then lift your other leg with the knee bent ninety degrees. Keep your arms at your sides for stabilization.

    Slowly, extend one leg out about half way, tap the big toe to the floor, then return to the starting position. Then extend the other leg out about half way, tap the big toe to the floor. Repeat these movements 6–12x.

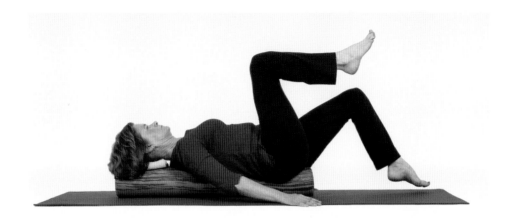

Note: *If you lose connection to the Core Hug—you will know this if you feel your low back come off the floor/roller—STOP. This means you are not ready. Go back to Step c, Standing, and practice until you are more stable.*

    If you can complete *all* the previous steps without your low back coming off the floor/roller, try these advanced steps.

2.   With the Core Hug fully engaged, extend your right leg fully, so it is parallel to the floor, with the foot flexed. Keep your left leg bent at ninety degrees. Arms are on the floor at your sides for stabilization.

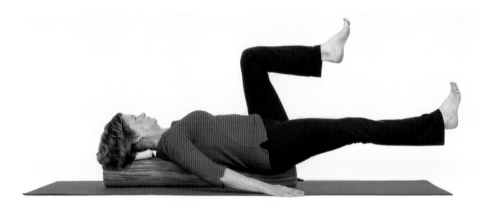

    Return to the starting position with both knees up and bent at ninety degrees.

    Repeat on the left side: Extend your left leg fully, so it is parallel to the floor, with the foot flexed and your other leg bent at ninety degrees. Keep your arms on the floor at your sides.

    Repeat on both sides four to six times.

Note: *Be sure your low back does not come off the roller or the floor. If it does, go back to the previous step.*

Advanced: If you can maintain full stability throughout this last step, you can move onto this advanced step. While extending one leg out as in Step 2, extend the opposite arm straight up over your head. Keep the other arm on the floor as a stabilizer. Most of the stabilization should come from the Core Hug and the Vertical Core.

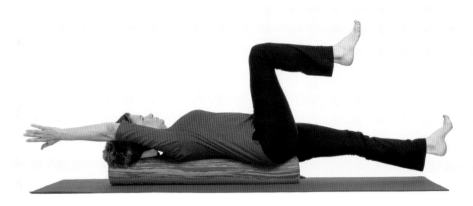

Repeat on the opposite side, switching arms and legs. Repeat four to six times, switching sides as if walking.

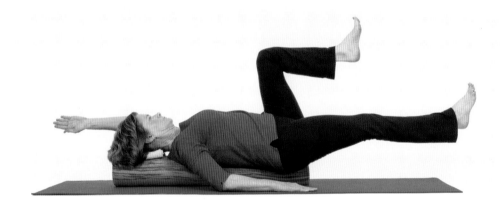

Stop, rest, feel the signals pulsating through your Core Hug and Vertical Core.

11. Coming Off the Roller

(intermediate, advanced)
Goals: To come off the roller safely and mindfully.
To sustain correct alignment once off the roller.

Bring your arms and legs back to starting position, with your feet on floor, hips-width apart. Slowly come off the roller by placing your hands on the floor, straightening out one leg, and sliding off that side—first your pelvis, then your torso, then your head.

12. Reassessing Your Alignment

(on the floor)

Goal: To take the time to feel the connections you have just made to the Core Hug and the Vertical Core.

Don't skip this step! It's important to feel the connections you have made in your body. Lie on the floor with your arms and legs straight and relaxed, palms up. Breathe slowly and take a few moments to feel the changes you have made in your alignment. Feel how your right and left sides are more balanced and more connected. Sense how the breath moves from your belly to your chest. The shoulders are more open, the neck more relaxed. Most of all, feel the connections to your Core Hug and your Vertical Core.

13. Opening Hip Fans on the Floor

(beginners/intermediate)

Goals: To melt the fascia in the front of the hips, the iliopsoas. This is the most important muscle in the body for posture, movement, and stability.

To reconnect the Vertical Core from the arches of the feet through the iliopsoas to the shoulders.

Lie on the floor. Fold your knees into your chest. Rock slowly side to side to relax the low back before beginning this exercise.

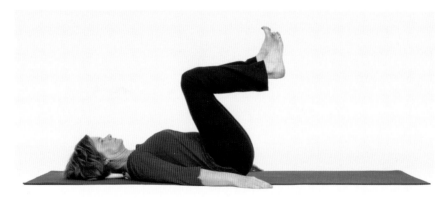

Place your right foot on the floor, right knee is bent. Straighten your left leg and left arm toward the ceiling.

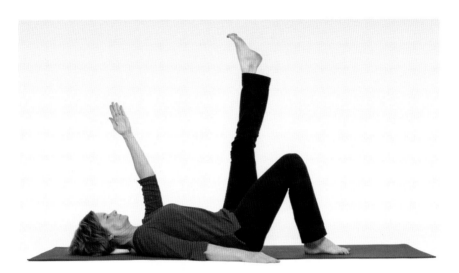

Reach your left leg and arm up to the ceiling to open the hip and shoulder joints. Extend your left leg away from you, reaching out of the hip joint. Extend your left arm up over your head, reaching out of the shoulder joint. Reach long!

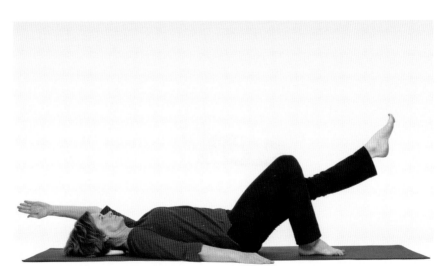

When your left heel touches the floor, flex the foot strongly. Reach the leg out of the hip. When your left hand touches the floor, grab the left wrist with your right hand to reach out of the shoulder. Feel the full body extension. With your left foot flexed, turn the foot out and push the heel of the left foot away from you. Activate the connection of the Vertical Core from the arch to the shoulder. Release. Then reach the foot and hand and activate the connections again. Release. Reach out, release. Repeat two to three times. As you reach long, feel the connections all through the body.

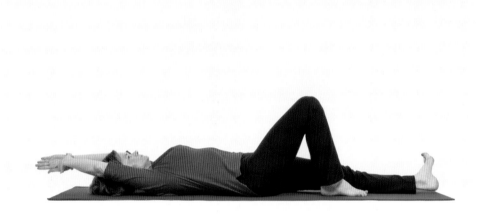

To strengthen the connection, with your body in full extension, keep the left foot turned out and, continuing to reach long, lift your left leg up about one-half inch off the floor, then release it down. Repeat this up and down movement four to six times. Connect to the strength within the body's Vertical Core.

Return to starting position. Notice the length on the side you stretched. Repeat the same sequence on the right side. Notice the length on this side.

14. Opening Hip Fans on the Roller

(advanced only)

If you are advanced, you may do this exercise on the roller as pictured below. Turn the roller horizontally and put it under your pelvis. Place it across the sacroiliac joints at the base of the spine (not under the low back) as pictured. Make sure you feel the natural sink and scoop of the pelvis (don't arch the back or tuck your pelvis under; this should be a relaxed position). Make sure you have been practicing the Core Hug and the Vertical Core training consistently before you attempt this on the roller.

Follow the same directions as exercise 13, but on the roller: Fold your knees into your chest. Rock side to side to relax the low back before beginning this exercise. Place one foot on the floor, knee bent. Straighten the opposite leg and arm toward the ceiling.

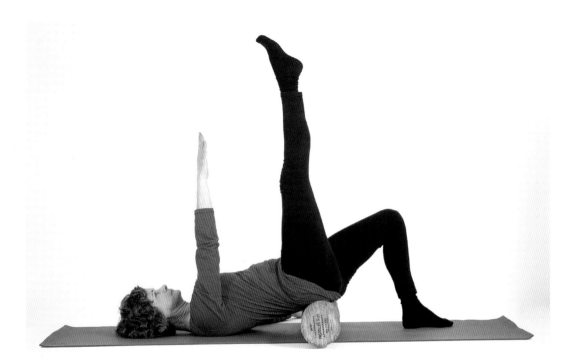

Reach your leg and arm up toward the ceiling to open the hip and shoulder joints. Extend your leg away from you, reaching out of the hip joint. Extend your arm up over your head, reaching out of the shoulder joint. Reach long!

When your heel touches the floor, flex the foot strongly. Reach the leg out of the hip. When your hand touches the floor, grab the wrist with your opposite hand to reach out of the shoulder. Feel the full body extension. With your foot flexed, turn the foot out and push the heel of the foot away from you. Activate the connection of the Vertical Core from the arch to the shoulder. Release. Then reach the foot and hand and activate the connections again. Release. Reach out, release. Repeat two to three times. As you reach long, feel the connections all through the body.

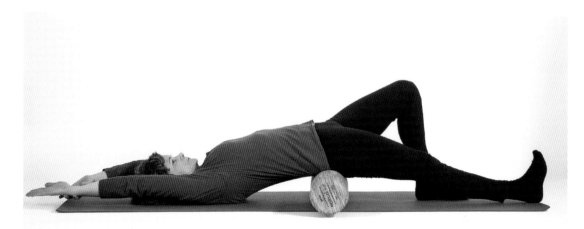

To strengthen the connection, with your body in full extension, keep your foot turned out and, continuing to reach long, lift your leg up about one-half inch off the floor then release down. Repeat this up and down movement four to six times. Connect to the strength within the body's Vertical core.

Return to starting position. Notice the length on the side you stretched. Repeat the same sequence on the other side. Notice the length on this side.

15. Block Hug (optional)

(all levels on the floor)
Goal: To quickly and efficiently connect the Core Hug and the Vertical Core.
Materials needed: two yoga blocks or Pilates rings

This exercise can be done as a quick way to connect the Core Hug and the Vertical Core. If you don't have time to do the whole routine, this is a good exercise to do to make the deep inner core connections needed for sitting, standing, and walking.

Lie on your back with your knees bent and your feet hips-width apart.

Place a yoga block or Pilates ring comfortably between your inner thigh fans. Using subtle activation movements, gently press your feet (about 3 ounces of pressure) into the floor, then gently press the block between your thighs. Notice that the Core Hug activates naturally. Repeat these steps slowly and with awareness four to six times. Feel the arches of the feet connecting up through the inseam of your legs, through the inner thigh fans, and into the body's center of gravity.

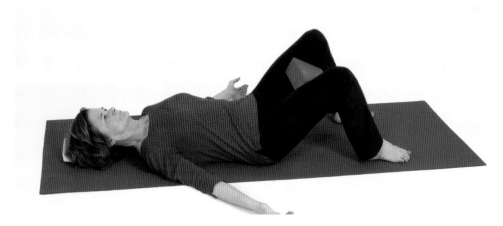

Bend your elbows and place them so they softly hug the side of your ribs. Hold a second yoga block between your hands with your fingers pointed toward the ceiling. Widen and spread your shoulder fans in front of your shoulders. Imagine you are holding a huge beach ball so your shoulders stay open and wide. Take a slow, deep inhalation, bringing the breath into the shore of your chest. As you exhale, press your elbows toward your feet, bring your shoulder blades (your back triangles) in and down toward your spine, gently press the block. Feel your shoulder girdle supported by the Core Hug and the Vertical Core. Repeat four to six times.

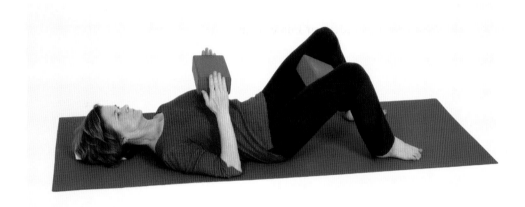

Now, put it all together. Gently press your feet into floor, then gently press the block between your thighs. Feel the Core Hug. Press your elbows toward your feet and the block between your hands. Feel the Core Hug and Vertical Core connected through your whole body!

A Note to Practitioners

No matter what method of bodywork or healing modality you practice—massage therapy, myofascial release, physical or occupational therapy, osteopathy, chiropractic, acupuncture, Zero Balancing, or Reiki—or what kind of movement education you provide—yoga, Pilates, fitness, core work, the Alexander Technique, Aston Kinetics, Somatic Education—the new anatomy of fascia and how it communicates throughout the body is important to know. Bodywork practitioners and movement educators can empower others to treat their own bodies with the awareness and self-care they deserve. In addition, learning about the inner core from this new paradigm can enhance what you already do. Giving yourself and your clients a user-friendly approach to aligning the body from the body's center of gravity and the inner core can enhance the work you do in the treatment room or in your classes or trainings.

It is especially important for fitness or movement educators to train their clients or students how to connect to the center of gravity with breath and activate the inner core *before* engaging in any exercise routine. This method can help prevent injury so people can keep moving and exercising as they age. Many knowledgeable and astute teachers have already begun teaching from the inner core and have noticed a profound difference. One excellent yoga teacher, Scott Anderson, creator of Alignment Yoga, begins each class with pre-yoga exercises to awaken and strengthen the inner core muscles for postural support. Before going into the yoga poses, the inner core is activated.

If you are a bodyworker, movement educator, or health care practitioner, please feel free to contact me at karen@gablersustainablebody.com. You can also visit my website, www.gablersustainablebody.com, for more information. I am willing to share the Sustainable Body hands-on and/or movement training so you can move your clients and students forward into core connection and stabilization. This method can enhance and complement any modality that you practice.

Conclusion:
A Better Way Forward

Foreman ends her book, *A Nation in Pain*, with the powerful claim that pain care is "a fundamental human right" and that we have "a moral imperative" to address the treatment of pain.[63] Every day, I meet people with chronic pain, and I see how much they suffer. Many have sought help and tried many treatments without success. They have exhausted their resources and feel hopeless that they will never be free of pain.

Foreman calls for "a true cultural transformation in the way pain is viewed and treated."[64] I believe this transformation starts with understanding the root causes of pain I have outlined in this book. We need to embrace the importance of the tensional fascial network in the human body and how understanding fascia may help us develop more effective methods for treating chronic pain. We need to educate doctors and medical educators about how some of the answers to chronic pain lie in the fascia. Studies have found that we can restore balance within the body down to the cellular level using our continuous fascial network. As I mentioned earlier, science is documenting that mechanics-driven or hands-on therapies could one day replace or enhance drug-based treatments for pain.[65] When we better understand why chronic pain *actually* happens, we can begin to effectively treat it from the inside out.

The bodyworkers-turned-scientists of the Fascia Research Society continue to conduct studies on fascia, pain, movement, and treatments. Through their research, we are coming to a better understanding of where chronic pain comes from and how to treat it. This research is part of an ongoing cultural transformation. Because the medical industry has not caught up to much of this research, people living in chronic pain may

---

63 Foreman, Judy. (2014). *A Nation in Pain.* Oxford University Press. p. 300.
64 Foreman, Judy. (2014). *A Nation in Pain.* Oxford University Press. p. 306.
65 Ingber, Donald. 1998 Jan. The Architecture of Life. *Scientific American; 278:* 48–57. Retrieved from http://time.arts.ucla.edu/Talks/Barcelona/Arch_Life.htm

need to put together their "own program of healing—integrating the best of Western *and* complementary medicine."[66]

Developing your own program of healing begins with your body's brilliant design. By educating yourself about your body's architecture and how fascia connects this architecture within you, you will be able to access the natural alignment of your body. When you perform the Sustainable Body training routine with awareness, you will learn to embody this architecture from the inside out, so you are empowered to live a life without pain.

This self-empowerment is so important because many people experience an access barrier to self-care. They cannot afford yoga, Pilates, or barre classes. Expensive gym memberships and personal trainers are out of reach. They do not have access to private practitioners of complementary medicine, especially when many are not covered by health insurance. High-quality bodywork or movement education may not be available to them.

We do not have to spend thousands of dollars on external solutions to our pain. We do not have to put ourselves at the mercy of others and look outside ourselves for the answers to our pain. Ergonomic chairs, standing desks, expensive pillows and mattresses—most are only temporary relief from deeper issues in the body. We do not have to depend on doctors, prescription drugs, or surgeries to fix what is broken. We do not have to blame our family history of bad backs or poor posture for our chronic pain. We do not have to blame our job or our partner for creating our stress. We do not have to injure ourselves when we exercise.

Instead of looking for the answers outside of ourselves and for other people to fix us, there is a way to be free from chronic pain from the inside. You are not destined to a life of chronic pain; your architecture is designed to keep you out of pain. The human body is organized in an intelligent way to stabilize and move from the center of gravity and the Vertical Core. When we use this intelligent design well, the body can heal itself from chronic pain and injury. In fact, it is designed so well that you have the architecture within your fascia and your bones to create alignment, balance, and to bounce back from the stresses and strains of life.

---

66 Foreman, Judy. (2014). *A Nation in Pain.* Oxford University Press. p.306.

Your fascia and your bones are designed to hold you up in alignment and suspension using a minimal amount of energy. Your fascia is designed to give you power and strength. Your fascia loves to communicate within its fluid, dynamic system if you keep it aligned and hydrated. Using your tools of mindful attention, you can reclaim this architecture.

We *do* have the power within us to treat our chronic pain. If we take the time to listen to the wisdom living in our bones and flesh, there is an avenue of treatment. By taking the time to explore and to be aware, to breathe the way we are meant to breathe, and to reconnect to the center of gravity and the inner core, we can change the alignment and movement codes within the body's internet. We can rebalance, reset, and revitalize the neurofascial system no matter what age we are, what level of fitness, or what stage of chronic pain we are in. We each deserve to find a path toward healing. It takes empowering ourselves with the knowledge of the brilliant design that lies within our bodies. The design is there. Let's embody it today and begin the journey of living an aligned, empowered, and pain-free life.

Acknowledgments

I am deeply grateful to my literary agent, Danielle Burby, whose enthusiasm, belief in my voice, and grounding support have been instrumental in my first foray into writing a book. Thank you for going above and beyond in every single way, Danielle.

I want to thank Brooke and Abigail at Skyhorse Publishing, who took a chance on this project. Thank you for respecting my vision and believing in this work. I am forever grateful.

I want to thank Tom Myers for introducing me to the new anatomy of fascia and for his innovative work in mapping the fascial web. Tom, your perspective opened my eyes to a new paradigm of looking at the body, without which this book would not exist. Thank you also to Yaron Gal Carmel for adding to my understanding of the deep inner core. With the two of you, I was able to bring it all together in a new way.

Deep gratitude also goes to Dr. Fritz Smith, the creator of Zero Balancing. Without Fritz's knowledge of bone and energy and how to balance the structural and energetic inner core, I would not have evolved my method. Another deeply felt gratitude goes to Jim McCormick, my Zero Balancing teacher, mentor, colleague, and friend. Without Jim, I would not have delved so deeply into the study of Zero Balancing nor experienced the profound healing that occurs through balancing the body's inner core.

I will always be thankful to Lakshmana Estabrooks, my first teacher in fascia and Structural Integration. She mentored me into the world of fascia and Structural Integration for the first ten years of my career as a bodyworker and movement educator. Her knowledge and expertise laid the foundation for my work in the fascial system.

I would also like to acknowledge Judith Aston, my movement teacher, for the biomechanical genius that she is. Judith taught me the basic concepts of movement and alignment from the inside and that posture does not come from the outside.

I will always have gratitude for my first yoga teacher, Patricia Walden, who is now a renowned teacher of Iyengar Yoga. I also thank another excellent yoga teacher, Carol Nelson. These Iyengar Yoga teachers extraordinaire laid the foundation for my alignment through a strong practice of yoga from the inside out.

I also want to thank the extraordinary masters and pioneers in the field of bodywork and movement who have influenced me: Robert Schleip, director of the Fascia Research Project, and Divo Müller, who together created Fascial Fitness; Gil Hedley; Mary Bond; F. M. Alexander; Sharon Wheeler; JoAnn Staugaard-Jones; Adjo Zorn; John Barns; Denise Deig of Positional Release Technique; Eric Franklin for his contributions to the world of somatic education, guided imagery, and movement principles; and Sue Hitzmann for bringing awareness of the importance of fascia to a wider audience.

I want to thank Ralph Taylor, my client and philanthropist of the highest caliber, who helped me bring my work out into the world. And to Fran West, whose belief in my work and innate generosity continually encourage me.

Special thanks to Bill Bowman of Bowman Design and Direction, my creative director extraordinaire. He dedicated his expertise and skill to rebrand and get my work out into the cyberworld. Thanks to Bill, my domains are secured, and my brand, website, marketing materials, and photographs reflect the essence of my work. For Bill's dedication to my work and to his generosity, I am eternally grateful.

I also want to thank my talented illustrator, Chiara Pieri, who called on her artistic skills to capture the new anatomy of fascia. Her dedication and enthusiasm for my work led to the imagery of fascia that makes its debut in this book.

I would like to express gratitude for the many clients who have worked with me over the last thirty-plus years, especially to those I worked with during the development of Sustainable Body over the last seventeen years. Your willingness to explore and actively participate in the process, share your experiences, and give me feedback is deeply appreciated. Without your encouragement and belief in me, Sustainable Body would not have evolved into what it is today. You know who you are and I could not have done it without you. Thank you Mary Dewart, Wallis Raemer, Linda Krouner, Paul Krouner, Stephanie Sonnabend, Gail Norcross, Peter Jenkins, and Deb Rosene, who have been supporting me since the beginning of my quest into the inner core.

I would also like to thank my family, friends, and colleagues who supported me throughout my career and especially through the evolution of my work: my sister, Deb Halle, who always supports me in whatever I am doing, and her beautiful family. Laura Hays, Roy Gottlieb, Eliza Mallouk, Jessica Kern, Bill Mueller, Catherine Fernbach, Cynthia

Wood, Tricia Duffy, Megan Grennan, Lou Benson, Lea Delacour, and Ted Bayne. Thanks for believing in me. To Joy Fay, my boot camp instructor, who believed in my work and encouraged her fitness instructors and yoga teachers to take my classes. Dr. Angel Gangoy, my orthodontist, who weathered the storm of aligning my teeth so graciously. Gratefulness to Michelle and Gerry Magid for their constant support. Thank you to Anne Noonan, who believed in me and gave me writing tips when writing felt overwhelming. A deep thank you to Irving Kirsch, who offered two brilliant ideas for the book that I am grateful to have been able to incorporate before going to print. My friend, Trudy Seidman, who kept calling to check in to see how the writing was going and reminded me of how proud she is of me.

Lastly, and most importantly, I want to thank my daughter, Katherine, who has been by my side throughout. This book would not have manifested without her insight, support, editing skills, technical expertise, and love for me and for the essence of this work. She understands who I am and what I want to express, and she supports me in making this happen. Katherine, you know I could not have done this without you. You are part of my inner core and always will be. I love you from the inside out!

About the Author

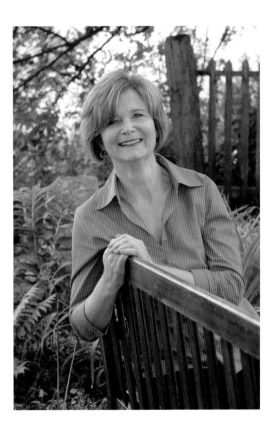

Karen M. Gabler is a Structural Integrator, Zero Balancer, Fascial Fitness instructor, movement educator, and licensed massage therapist, nationally certified in therapeutic massage and bodywork.

Her thirty-plus years of private practice, research, and study in complementary alternative medicine and movement education have culminated in the creation of Sustainable Body, a revolutionary approach to align and balance the body to live pain-free. She maintains a private practice and teaches her method to clients, practitioners, and movement instructors. Find out more at www.gablersustainablebody.com. Karen lives outside of Boston, Massachusetts.

References

Ament, R., R. Callahan, M. McClure, M. Reuling, and G. Tabor. 2014. Wildlife Connectivity: Fundamentals for conservation action. Center for Large Landscape Conservation: Bozeman, Montana. http://largelandscapes.org/media/publications/Wildlife-Connectivity-Fundamentals-for-Conservation-Action.pdf

Aston, Judith. 2007. *Moving Beyond Posture: In Your Body on the Earth.* Judith Aston.

Bond, Mary. 2006. *The New Rules of Posture: How to Sit, Stand, and Move in the Modern World.* Rochester, VT: Healing Arts Press.

Calais-Germain, Blandine. 2006. *Anatomy of Breathing.* Seattle, WA: Eastland Press.

Carmel, Yaron Gal. 2014. *The Deep Back Line and a Proposed Alternate Superficial Back Line.* International Association of Structural Integrators Yearbook.

Carter, S. and Porges, Stephen. 2013. *Evolution, Early Experience and Human Development.* New York, NY: Oxford University Press.

Claxton, Guy. (2015). *Intelligence in the Flesh: Why your mind needs your body much more than it thinks.* Yale University Press.

Earls, James, and Myers, Thomas. 2010. *Fascial Release for Structural Balance.* Berkeley, CA: North Atlantic Books.

Earls, James. 2014. *Born to Walk: Myofascial efficiency and the body in movement.* Berkeley, CA: North Atlantic Books.

Edwards, Michaelle. 2011. *YogAlign: Pain-Free Yoga from Your Inner Core.* Hihimanu Press.

Fascial Fitness Association. http://www.fascial-fitness.de/en/fascial-fitness

Foreman, Judy. 2014. *A Nation in Pain.* New York, NY: Oxford University Press.

Franklin, Eric. 2002. *Pelvic Power: Mind/body exercises for strength, flexibility, posture, and balance.* Hightstown, NJ: Elysian Editions.

Franklin, Eric. 2012. *Dynamic Alignment Through Imagery,* 2nd ed. Champaign, IL: Human Kinetics.

Gangemi, Stephen. http://sock-doc.com/natural-movement/ and http://www.drgangemi.com/natural-fitness/

Guimberteau, Jean-Claude. 2015. *Architecture of Human Living Fascia.* Edinburgh: Handspring Publishing.

Hamwee, John. 1999. *Zero Balancing: Touching the energy of bone.* London: Frances Lincoln.

Hitzmann, Sue. 2013. *The MELT Method: A Breakthrough Self-Treatment System to Eliminate Chronic Pain, Erase the Signs of Aging, and Feel Fantastic in Just 10 Minutes a Day!* New York, NY: Harper Collins.

Ho, Mae-Wan, and White, David P. The Acupuncture System and The Liquid Crystalline Collagen Fibers of the Connective Tissues. American Journal of Complementary Medicine (in press). Institute of Science in Society http://www.i-sis.org.uk/lcm.php.

Ingber, Donald. 1998 Jan. The Architecture of Life. *Scientific American; 278:* 48–57. Retrieved from http://time.arts.ucla.edu/Talks/Barcelona/Arch_Life.htm

Levin, Stephen M. 2016. http://biotensegrity.com/

Lyon, Bret. (2012 Jan 14). Anatomy of a Freeze - or Dorsal Vagal Shutdown. Retrieved from http://eiriu-eolas.org/2012/01/17/anatomy-of-a-freeze-or-dorsal-vagal-shutdown/

Myers, Thomas. 2014. *Anatomy Trains: Myofascial Meridians for Manual and Movement Therapists, 3rd Edition,* Churchill Livingstone.

Myers, Thomas. (2011, Mar 23). Fascial Fitness: Training in the NeuroMyofascial Web. *IDEA Fitness Journal, 8*(4). Retrieved from http://www.ideafit.com/fitness-library/fascial-fitness

Oschman, James L., Ph.D. *Readings on the Scientific Basis of Bodywork and Movement Therapies.* www.somatics.de

Scarr, Graham. 2014. *Biotensegrity: The Structural Basis of Life.* Handspring Publishing.

Schleip, Robert, Findley, Thomas W., Chaitow, Leon, and Huijing, Peter A. 2012. *Fascia: The Tensional Network of the Human Body.* Elsevier, Churchill Livingstone.

Schleip, Robert (ed.). 2015. *Fascia in Sport and Movement.* East London: Handspring Publishers.

Schultz, R. Louis, & Feitis, Rosemary. 1996. *The Endless Web: Fascial anatomy and physical reality.* Berkeley, CA: North Atlantic Books.

Smith, Fritz Frederick, MD. 1986. *Inner Bridges: A Guide to Energy Movement and Body Structure*. Atlanta, GA: Humanics Limited.

Smith, Fritz Frederick, MD. 2005. *Alchemy of Touch: Moving through mastery through the lens of Zero Balancing.* Taos, NM: Complementary Medicine Press.

Staugaard-Jones, JoAnn. 2012. *The Vital Psoas Muscle: Connecting Physical, Emotional, and Spiritual Well-Being.* Berkeley, CA: North Atlantic Books.

Townsend, Patty. 2016 Jul 14. Embodied Tensegrity, Fascia, and Yoga. Embodyogablog. com. Retrieved from https://embodyogablog.com/2016/07/14/embodied-tensegrity-fascia-and-yoga/.

Vranich, Belisa. 2014. *Breathe: 14 days to oxygenating, recharging, and fueling your body & brain.* New York, NY: Breathing Class Press.

Index

Page references in italics indicate a photo or illustration.